time in India. He reported role of cell mediated immunity in [illegible] calves. His pioneer work includes immunopathology due to pesticides, heavy metals, mycotoxins and nanoparticles. Dr. Chauhan developed a new method using MTT dye for detection of CMI responses. He has scientifically validated Panchgavya and named it as "Cowpathy".

He have been engaged internationally as Visiting Professor, University of Copenhagen and Advisor, WHO. Dr. Chauhan guided more than 50 scholars for Master's and Doctoral research; most of them are placed as Professors, Scientists, officers in Indian Army, banks and industry in India and abroad. At present he is working as Head Veterinary Pathology, Chairman Scientific Advisory Committee, ICMR-NARFBR, Member AWBI and CPCSEA (Govt of India). Prof Chauhan superannuated on 30th June 2024 after distinguish service of 41.5 years and still contributing to the profession through lectures, writings and research and meticulously developing (genuine) book for the benefit of students and young generation.

Dr. Deepak [illegible] Veterinary [illegible] Graduate in Veterinary Pathology from College of [illegible] Animal Sciences [illegible] and Technology [illegible] 2019 and 2020. He was awarded outstanding student award by [illegible] He visited [illegible] to present research paper in World poultry congress 2008. He joined [illegible]

[illegible] Under Graduate students. Dr. [illegible] awarded Young Scientist award by Society of Immunology and Immunopathology, Prakash best poster award, best paper presentation award by Indian Society of Veterinary Anatomy, best poster award by [illegible] Society of Veterinary [illegible] in National Conference held at ANDUA&T, Kumarganj, Ayodhya, Uttar Pradesh, India.

Systemic Veterinary Pathology

R.S. Chauhan
M.V.Sc., Ph.D. (Path.), FNAVS, FSIIP, FIAVP, PDCR, OCTT, ACPPM, MBA
(Ex- Advisor WHO, Ex- Director IVRI, Ex-JDCADRAD, Ex-Director IBT,
Ex- National Fellow ICAR)
Member Animal Welfare Board of India (Govt. of India)
Member, CCSEA (Govt of India)
Chairman, SAC, NARFBR (ICMR)
Ex-Professor and Head, Department of Veterinary Pathology
GB Pant University of Agriculture & Technology Pantnagar - 263 145
Uttarakhand, India

Desh Deepak Singh
M.V.Sc., Ph.D.
Professor and Head
Department of Veterinary Pathology
U. P. Pandit Deen Dayal Upadhyaya Pashu Chikitsa Vigyan Vishwavidyalaya Evam
Go Anusandhan, Sansthan (DUVASU), Mathura-281001, Uttar Pradesh, India

nipa®

NIPA® GENX ELECTRONIC RESOURCES & SOLUTIONS P. LTD.
New Delhi-110 034

NIPA® GENX ELECTRONIC
RESOURCES & SOLUTIONS P. LTD.
101,103, Vikas Surya Plaza, CU Block
L.S.C.Market, Pitam Pura, New Delhi-110 034
Ph : +91 11 4386 0225, 9717133558, 9540816132
E-mail: newindiapublishingagency@gmail.com
Website: www.niparesources.com

Print ISBN 978-93-58872-50-7

ebook ISBN: 978-93-58877-78-6

Composed and Designed by NIPA®.

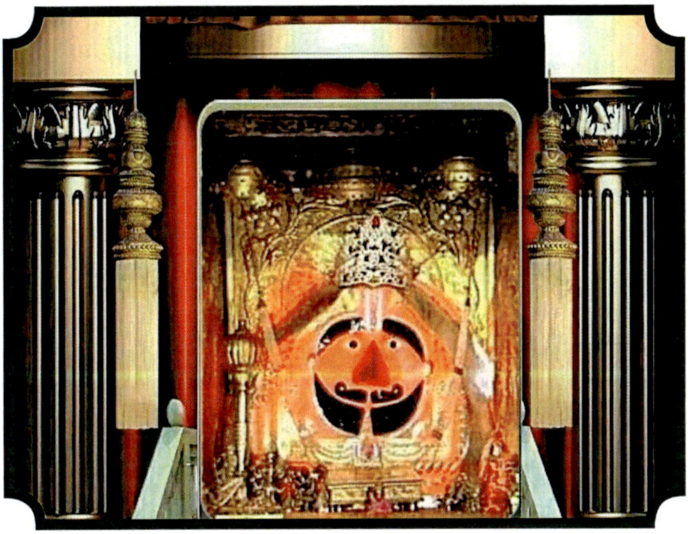

Dedicated to Anjani Nandan
Pavansut Lord Hanuman

Preface

Veterinary Pathology is an important discipline of Veterinary Sciences which makes a bridge in between the basic and clinical sciences. The knowledge of Veterinary Pathology makes the Veterinarian a perfect diagnostician particularly when his patients (animal) can't speak their illness to the doctor. Keeping in view the need of study of Veterinary Pathology to become a good Veterinary doctor, the book "Systemic Veterinary Pathology" is written for the use of teachers, students and field veterinarians. The complexity of the subject is presented in a simplified way particularly keeping the view of Indian geo-climatic conditions and animal population. However, students of Veterinary Science desire a compact text of Systemic Veterinary Pathology covering the VCI new syllabus of Pathology which can be utilized during their study and examinations particularly in competitive examinations. Hence, this textbook is prepared as a text material to all those who want to study Systemic Veterinary Pathology at undergraduate and postgraduate level and are interested in any kind of competitive examination or interview. It covers all the topics of Systemic Veterinary Pathology like Pathology of cutaneous system, musculoskeletal system, cardiovascular system, respiratory system, digestive system, hemopoietic and immune system, urinary system, genital system, nervous system, endocrine system, eyes and ear. The text is described in a very simple format including developmental as well as acquired pathological conditions in different body systems of animals and birds including their etiology, clinical manifestations, characteristic macroscopic and microscopic features along with diagnosis; only salient features are mentioned avoiding detailed text. Hope this book "Systemic Veterinary Pathology" not only will find a place in the young fraternity of Veterinary Science but also it will be highly useful to the field Veterinarians for diagnosing diseases on the basis of characteristic clinical manifestations, and lesions and in writing of post mortem report. The help rendered by our colleagues and students in preparation and designing of this book is duly acknowledged. Readers' comments are welcome to further improve the book.

R.S. Chauhan
D.D. Singh

Contents

1

Pathology of Cutaneous System

Developmental Anomalies

Congenital icthyosis

Congenital icthyosis is scaly epidermis which resembles the skin of fish and occurs due to a simple autosomal recessive homozygous gene in calves. This condition is characterized by scaly, horny, thick epidermis divided into plates by deep fissures. Microscopically, there is thick keratin layer over the epidermis (Fig.1.1).

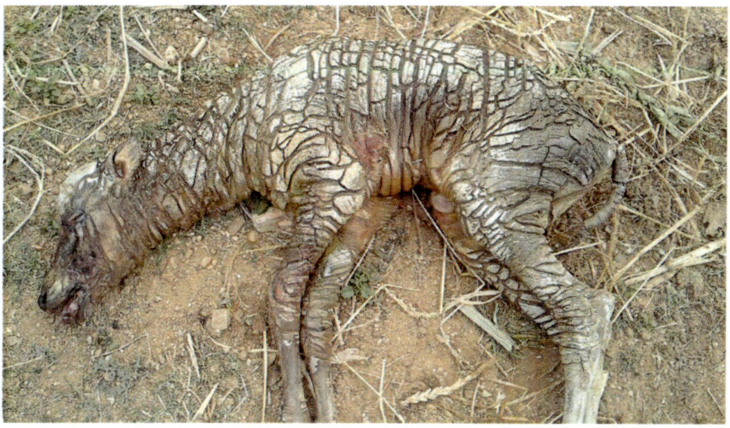

Fig 1.1: Congenital icthyosis

Epitheliogenesis imperfecta

Epitheliogenesis imperfecta is a congenital defect characterized by discontinuity of epithelium on skin leaving patches without squamous epithelium mostly at feet, claws and oral mucosa. Such defect may occur in calves which succumb to infection after birth or such foetus may abort. This disease condition is inherited as an autosomal recessive trait.

Congenital alopecia

Alopecia or hairlessness on the skin with complete lack of hair follicles has been observed in dog and other animals. Such hairless sites may follow a regular pattern or occurs in patches. This is a hereditary defect recognized in certain breeds.

Congenital albinism

Albinism is absence of melanin pigmentation due to deficiency of tyrosinase. This congenital abnormality is encountered sporadically due to a recessive trait in most species. The melanocytes are present but there is lack of melanin synthesis due to tyrosinase deficiency.

Congenital cutaneous asthenia

The collagen fibers are irregular in size and orientation and become fragmented due to disorganization of fibrils within the fibers. This condition occurs due to a deficiency in procollagen peptidase responsible for formation of collagen. This condition leads to hyper elasticity and fragility of skin and hypermotility of joints in cattle, sheep and dogs.

Acanthosis Nigricans

This is increased amount of melanin in skin along with hyperkeratosis. This condition commonly occurs in dogs, at ventral abdomen and medial surface of legs.

Etiology

- Hormonal imbalance.
- Tumors of testicles and pituitary gland.

Macroscopic features

- Colour of skin becomes black.
- Dry and scaly skin due to hyperkeratosis.

Microscopic features

- Proliferation of melanocytes and melanoblasts.
- Black/brown colour pigment intracellular/ extracellular.
- Cells appear as black or brown globular mass.

- Melanin granules are minute, dirty brown in colour and spherical in shape.
- Hyperkeratinization.

Dermatitis

Dermatitis is the inflammation of skin characterized by hyperemia, erythema, serus exudation and infiltration of neutrophils and mononuclear cells (Figs. 1.2 to 1.5).

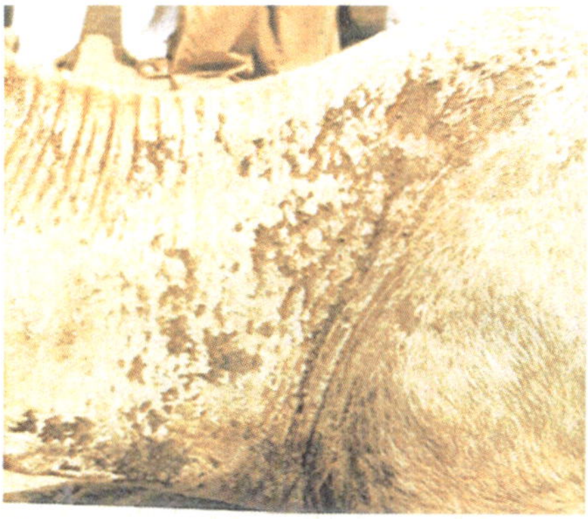

Fig. 1.2: Photograph of a camel showing skin patches of fungal dermatitis

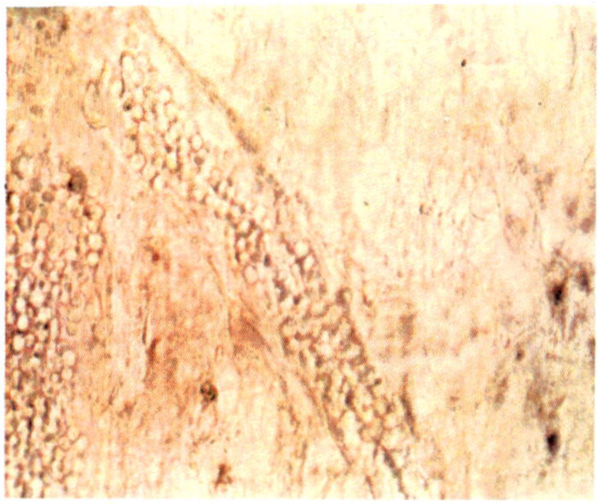

Fig. 1.3: Photomicrograph of skin scraping showing presence of fungus (*Trichophyton metagraphite*)

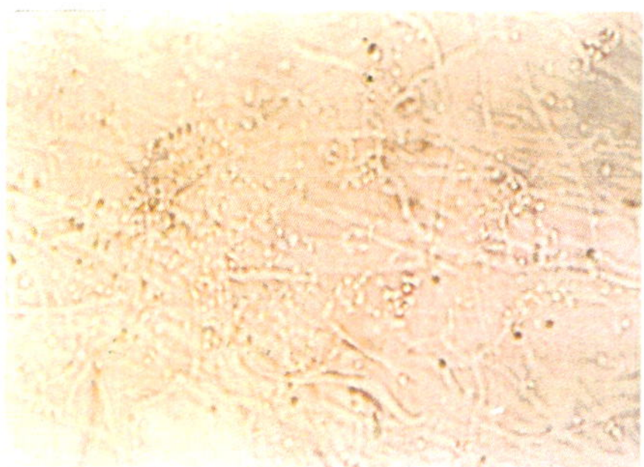

Fig. 1.4: Photomicrograph of skin scraping showing presence of fungus (*Trichophyton vericosum*)

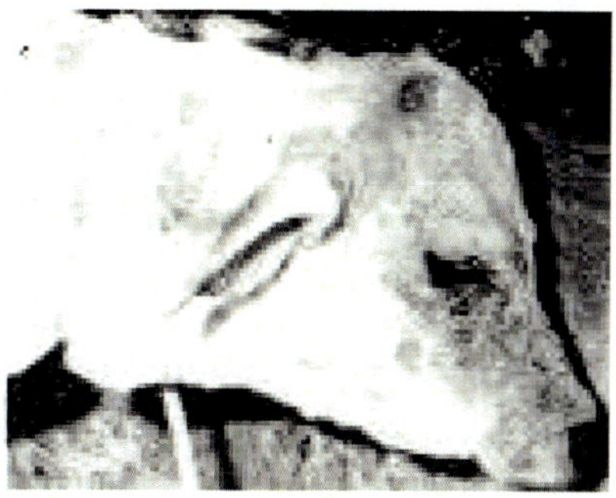

Fig. 1.5: Photograph of a calf showing ringworm on face

Etiology

- Bacteria, viruses, chemicals, allergy, trauma, fungi and their toxins.

Macroscopic features

- Erythematous patches on skin.
- Swelling of skin, itching sensation leads to damage/scratch due to rubbing.
- Loss of hairs, patches on skin, alopecia.

Microscopic features

- Hyperemia.
- Serus exudate.
- Infiltration of neutrophils and mononuclear cells.
- Presence of fungus in skin scrapings.

Vesicular Dermatitis

Vesicular dermatitis is excessive accumulation of clear fluid in dermis and epidermis leading to vesicle/blister formation. It is also known as hydropic dermatitis (Figs. 1.6 to 1.9).

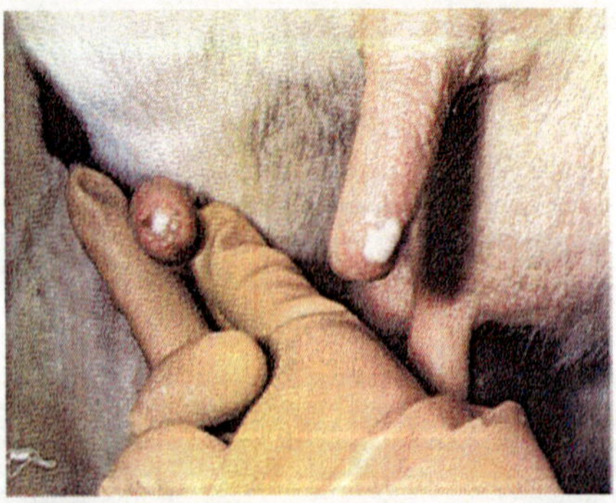

Fig. 1.6: Photograph showing vesicle on teat

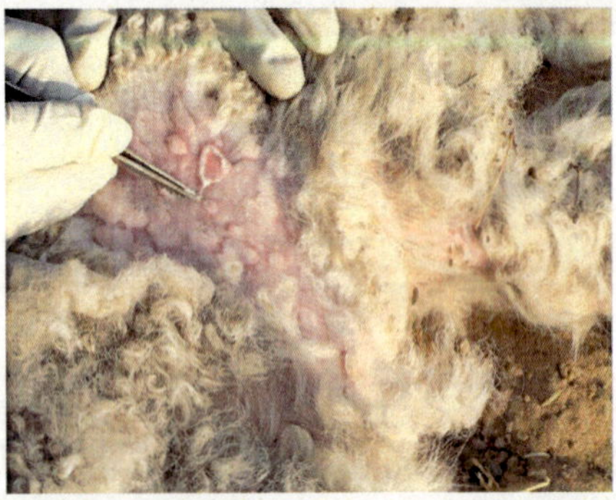

Fig. 1.7: Photograph showing vesicle on skin

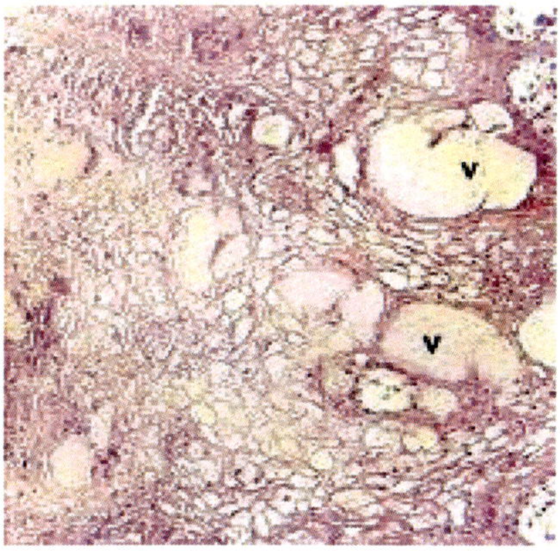

Fig 1.8: Photomicrograph showing hydropic degeneration and vesicle formation

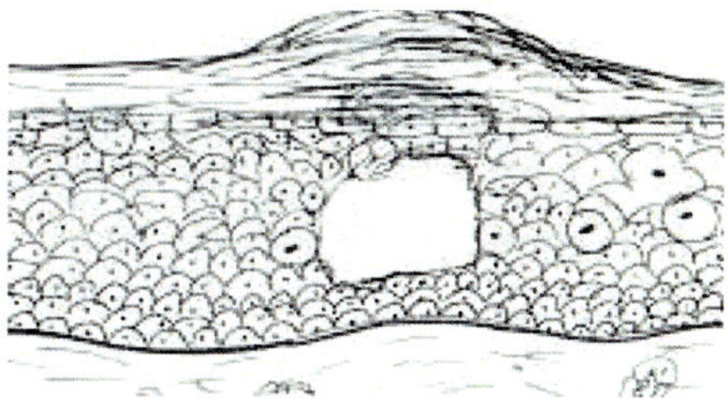

Fig. 1.9: Diagram of vesicle in skin

Etiology

- Sunburn.
- Heat.
- Foot and Mouth Disease virus.
- Pox virus.

Microscopic features

- Hyper keratinization of skin.
- Hyperemia
- Infiltration of neutrophils, lymphocytes, macrophages, eosinophils
- Presence of mites at the site of lesions

Allergic Dermatitis

This is the inflammation of skin sensitized to certain substances, known as allergens. Such inflammation can be seen as a result of delayed type hypersensitivity (DTH) reaction.

Macroscopic features

- Oedematous fluid in dermis and epidermis resulting in thickening of skin.
- Hyperemia, vesicles.
- Break of vesicles leads to clear fluid discharge.

Microscopic features

- Hyperemia.
- Accumulation of clear fluid in epidermis and dermis, which is characterized by clear spaces or takes light pink stain of eosin.
- Some cells show hydropic degeneration.
- Infiltration of leucocytes.

Parasitic Dermatitis (Acariasis)

Acariasis or mange is caused by mites and is characterized by hyperkeratosis and inflammation of skin leading to itching, rubbing and scratching (Figs. 1.10 to 1.19).

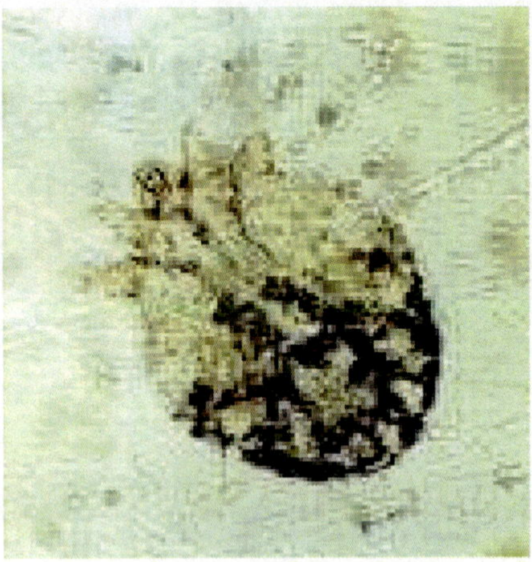

Fig. 1.10: Photomicrograph of *Sarcoptes scabei*

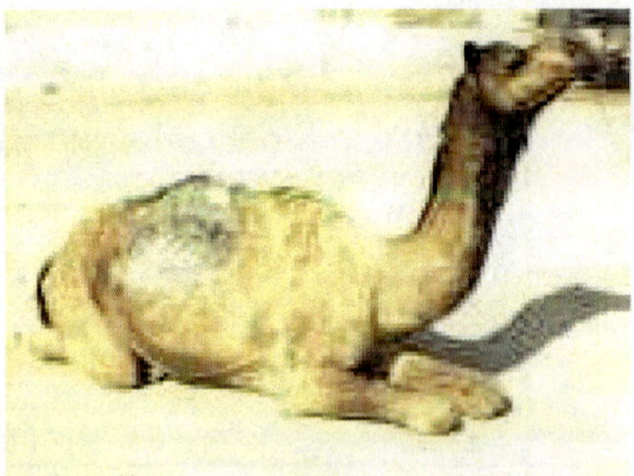

Fig. 1.11: Photograph showing mange due to *S. scabei* in a camel

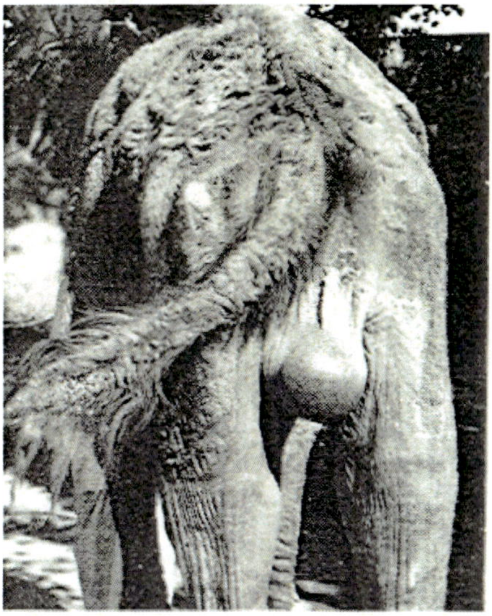

Fig. 1.12: Photograph of camel showing orchitis due to mange

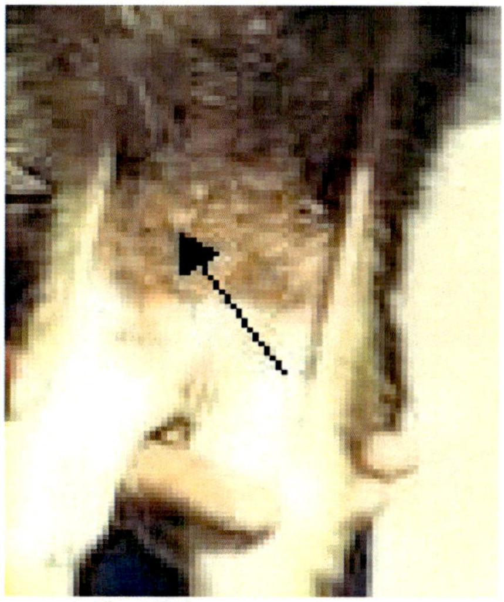

Fig. 1.13: Photograph of a dog showing pustular dermatitis due to demodectic mange

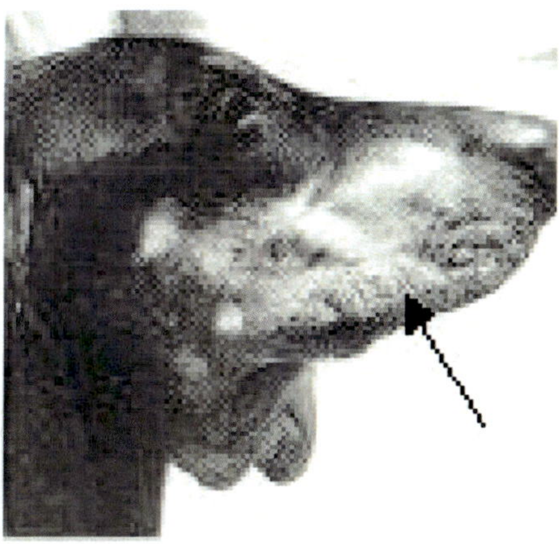

Fig. 1.14: Photograph of dog showing demodectic mange

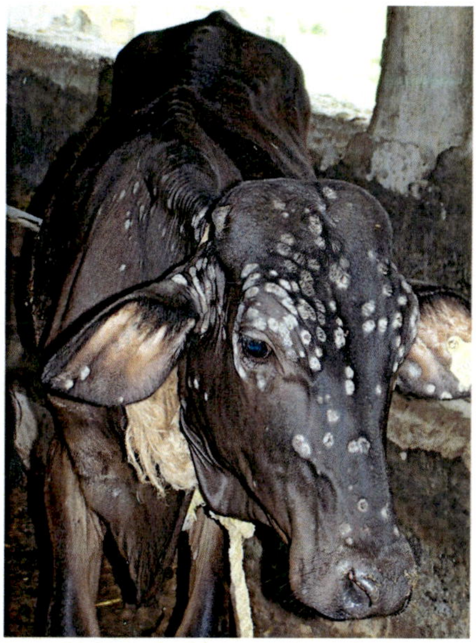

Fig. 1.15: Photograph of a cow showing demodectic mange.

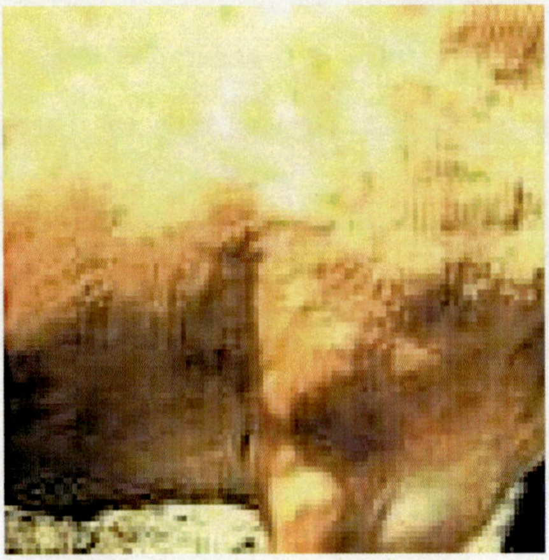

Fig. 1.16: Photograph of a cow showing. demodectic mange

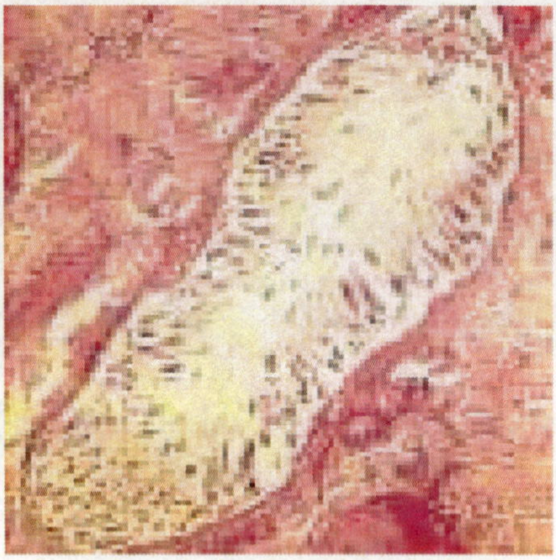

Fig. 1.17: Photomicrograph showing demodectic mites in cyst

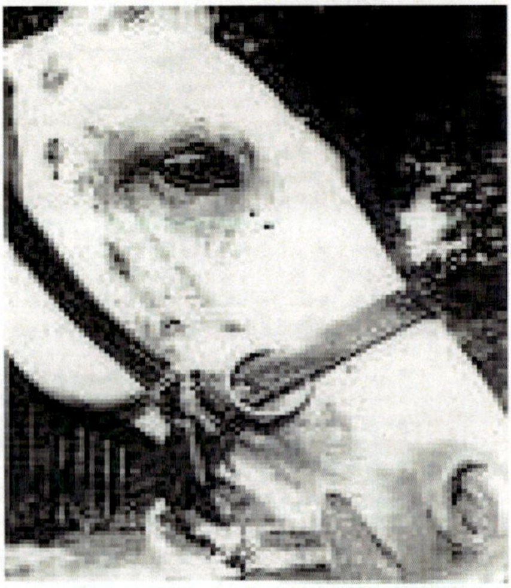

Fig. 1.18: Photograph of horse showing chorioptic mange

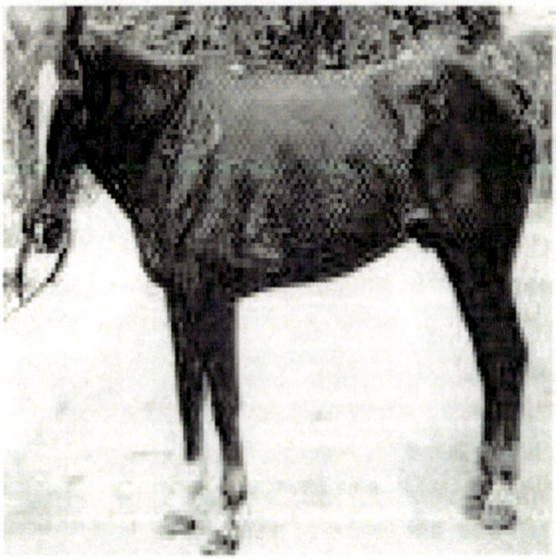

Fig. 1.19: Photograph of horse showing chorioptic mange

Etiology

• Mites

1. *Sarcoptes scabei*
2. *Psoroptic* sp.
3. *Demodectic* sp.
4. *Chorioptic* sp.

Macroscopic features

- Hyperkeratosis of skin, dry and scaly appearance of skin.
- Haemorrhage/trauma due to rubbing/ scratching as a result of intense itching.
- Absence of hairs on lesions.

Etiology

- Chemicals (DNCB/DNFB) (Figs.1.20 & 1.21).
- Tuberculin reaction (Figs. 1.22 & 1.23).
- Allergic reaction due to Lantana plants (Fig.1.24).
- Soaps, detergents, organic chemicals.
- Parasites- fleas.

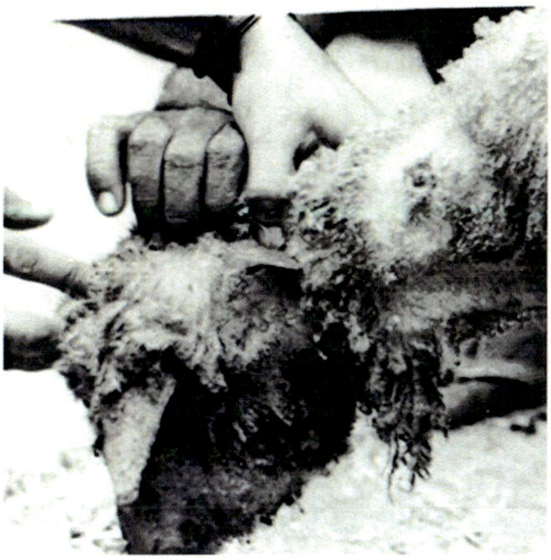

Fig. 1.20: Photograph of sheep showing DTH reaction

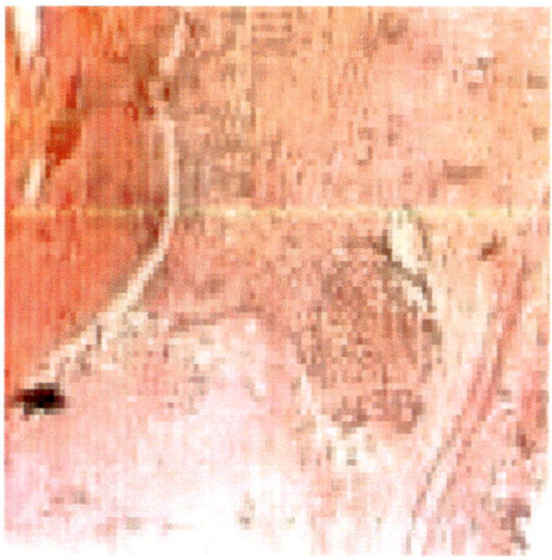

Fig 1.21: Photomicrograph showing DTH reaction in skin

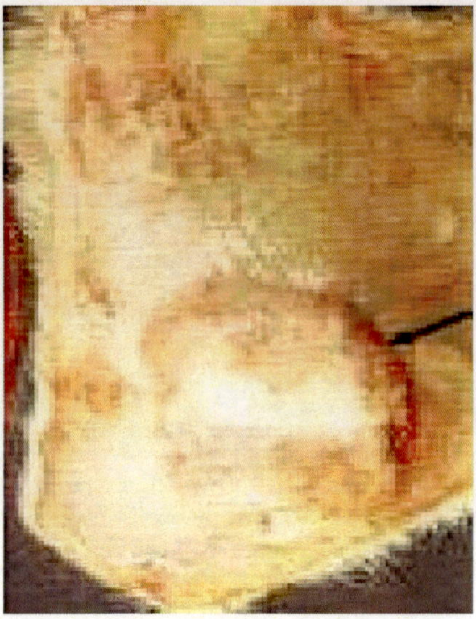

Fig. 1.22: Photograph of tuberculoid

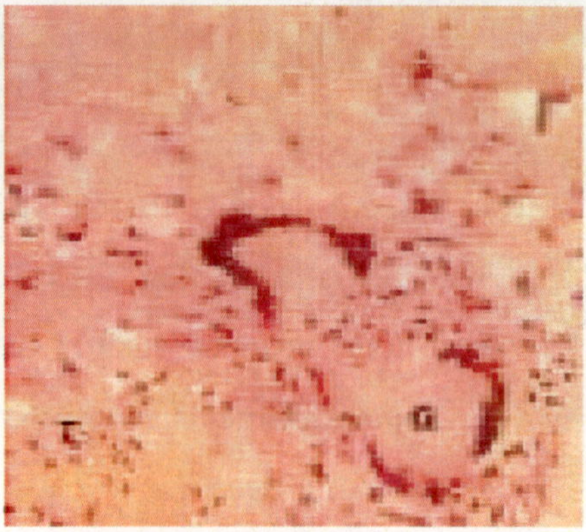

Fig. 1.23: Photomicrograph of tuberculoid dermatitis

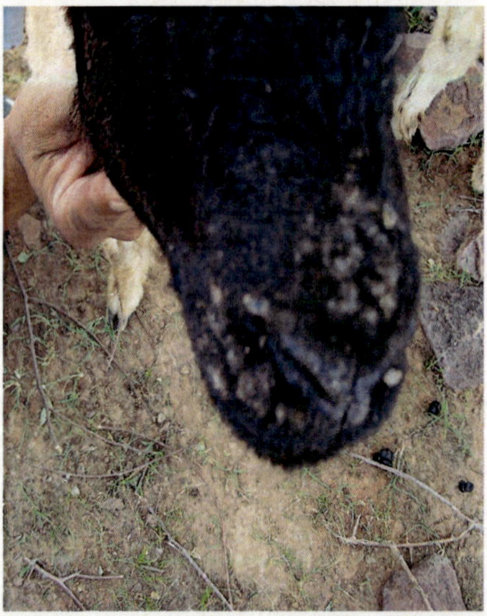

Fig. 1.24: Allergic reaction due to Lantana poisoning in sheep

Macroscopic features

- Hyperemia, erythema
- Oedematous/nodular swelling, hard to touch.

- Hot, painful.
- Atopy with vesicular rash, pruritus, serus exudate.

Microscopic features

- Infiltration of eosinophils and mononuclear cells, macrophages, lymphocytes.
- Hyperemia, oedema, necrosis.

Gangrenous Dermatitis

Gangrenous dermatitis is the inflammation of skin along with formation of gangrene caused by fungal toxins and characterized by sloughing of skin, dry gangrene with break in epidermis.

Etiology

- *Fusarium* sp. toxins
- Rice straw feeding – Degnala disease.

Macroscopic features

- Presence of gangrenous inflammation on extremities such as legs, udder, ears, tail, scrotum (Figs. 1.25 to 1.27).
- Sloughing of skin leaving raw surface.
- Sloughing of sp. hooves with hemorrhage.

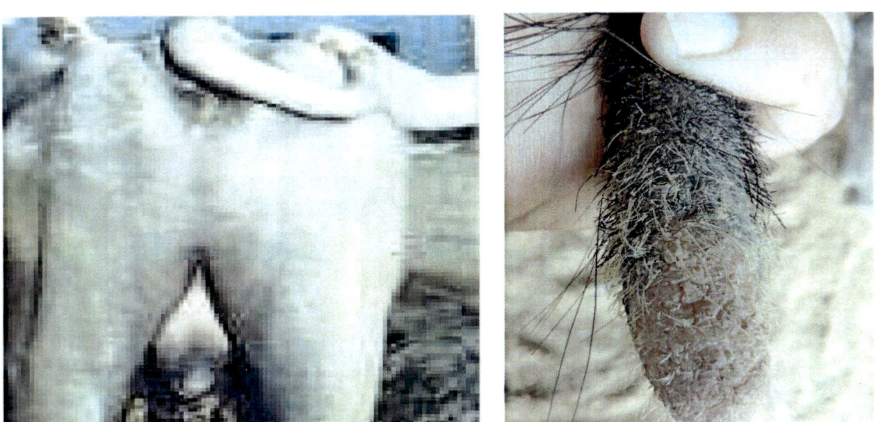

A B

Fig. 1.25: Photograph showing dry gangrene on scrotum (A) and tail (B) of a buffalo bull due to fusariotoxicosis

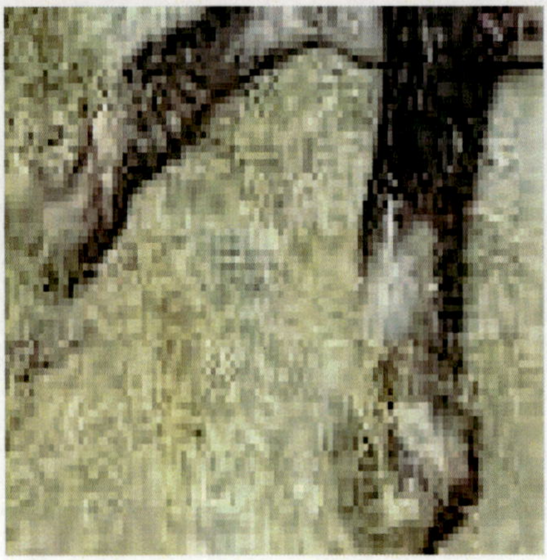

Fig. 1.26: Photograph showing sloughing of sp. hooves in buffalo due to fusariotoxicosis

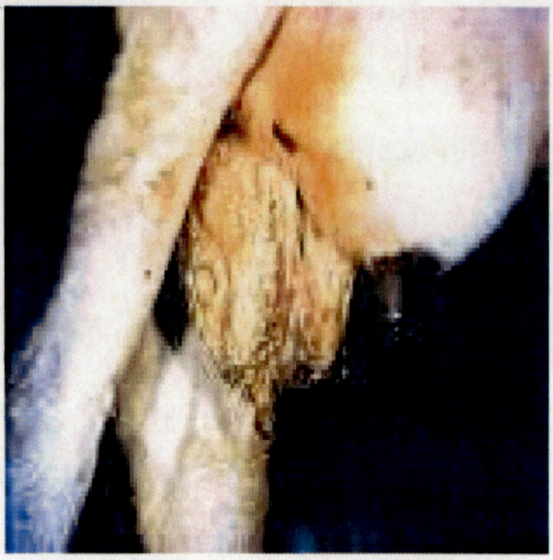

Fig. 1.27: Photograph showing sloughing of skin from udder due to fusariotoxicosis

Microscopic features

- Inflammation of skin and invasion by saprophytes causing dissolution of cells/tissue.
- Infiltration of mononuclear cells at the periphery of the lesion.

Equine Cutaneous Granuloma

There is development of chronic, ulcerated and on limb of horses due to wire cuts or other cutaneous injury.

Etiology

- Skin cuts/injury.
- Habronemiasis.
- Phycomycosis.
    - *Hyphomyces destruens*
    - *Entomorphthora coronata*

Macroscopic features

- Granulation of tissue in wound.
- Presence of yellowish/white specks.
- Summer sores/Bursatti.

Microscopic features

- Tissue composed of newly formed fibrous tissue, with large number of capillaries, infiltration of eosinophils.
- Presence of necrotic masses, stains deep red with H&E.
- Presence of helminths in section – cutaneous habronemiasis.
- Presence of septate hyphae of fungus.

Miscellaneous Lesions of Skin

Papule: Focal hyperplasia of stratum spinosum epithelium leading to hard nodular eruption on skin (Fig. 1.28).

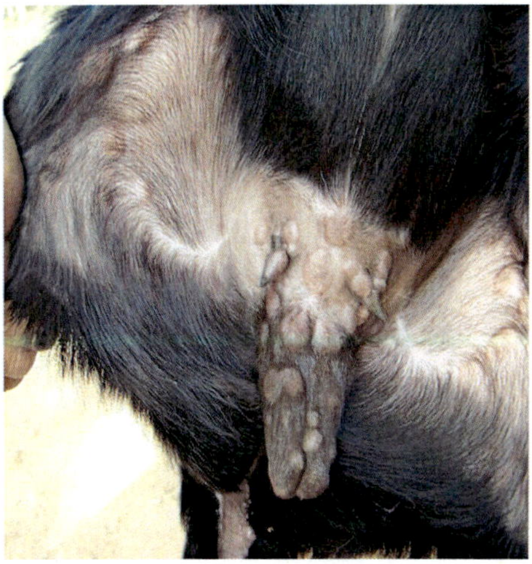

Fig. 1.28: Papules in Goat pox

Vesicle: A cavity in epidermis containing fluid and covered by a thin layer of epidermis elevated from the surface (Figs. 1.7, 1.8 and 1.9).

Pustule: A vesicle filled with pus (Fig. 1.13).

Scab: A dried papule / pustule (Fig. 1.29 to 1.32).

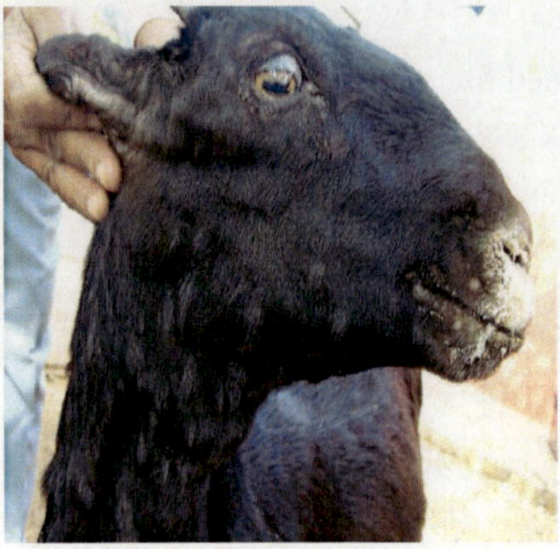

Fig. 1.29: Scab formation in skin – Goat pox

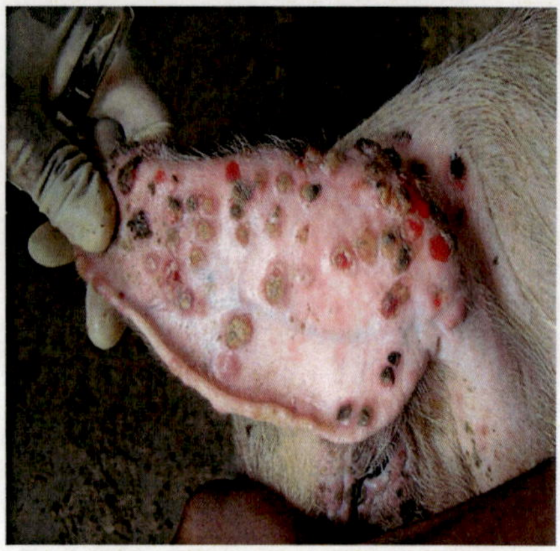

Fig. 1.30: Ear of pig showing pock lesions

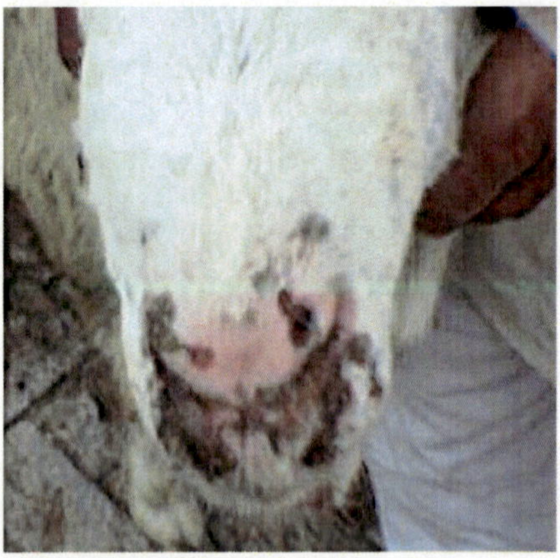

Fig. 1.31: Sheep mouth showing pock lesions

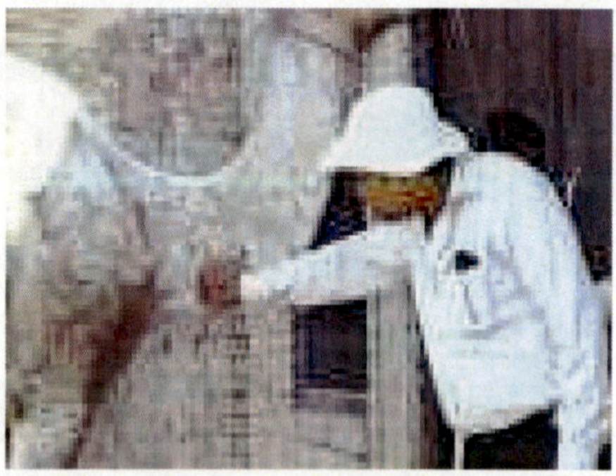

Fig. 1.32: Photograph showing presence of scab and scar on skin of camel.

Acanthosis: Thickening of epidermis due to hyperplasia of stratum spinosum/prickle cell layer (Fig. 1.33).

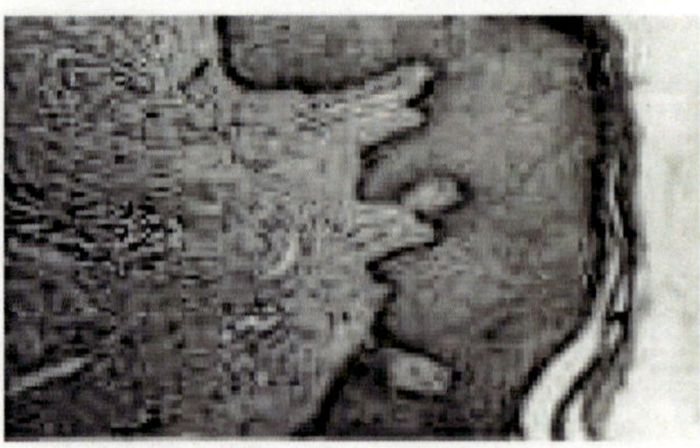

Fig. 1.33: Photomicrograph of skin showing Acanthosis

Hyperkeratosis: Thickening of keratin layer stratum corneum.

Parakeratosis: The retention of nucleus in keratin layer.

Bulla/bleb: Cavitations in epidermis filled with fluid and larger than vesicle.

Erosion/Excoriation: Superficial loss of epithelium (Fig. 1.34).

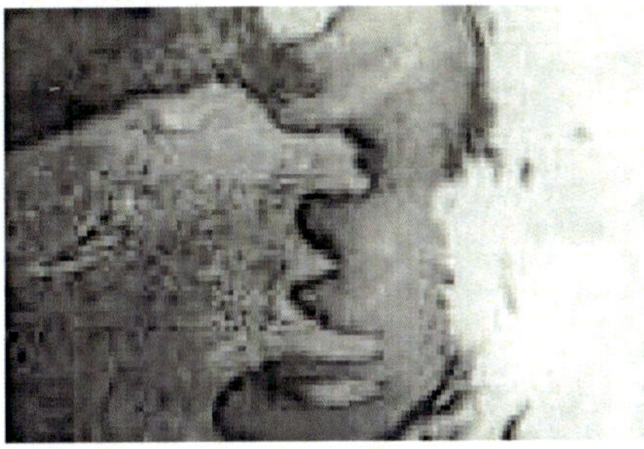

Fig. 1.34: Photomicrograph of skin showing erosion

Fissure: Linear defect in epidermis, which may be crusted at mucocutaneous junctions.

Abscess: A circumscribed cavity filled with pus (Fig.1.35).

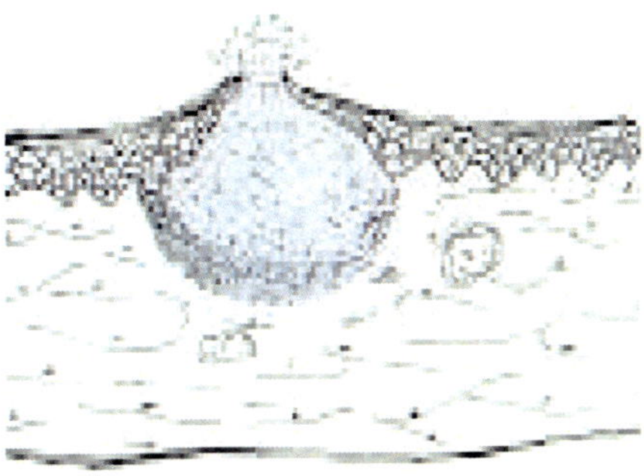

Fig. 1.35: Diagram of abscess

Ulcer: A break in the continuity of the epidermis exposing dermis (Fig. 1.36 & 1.37).

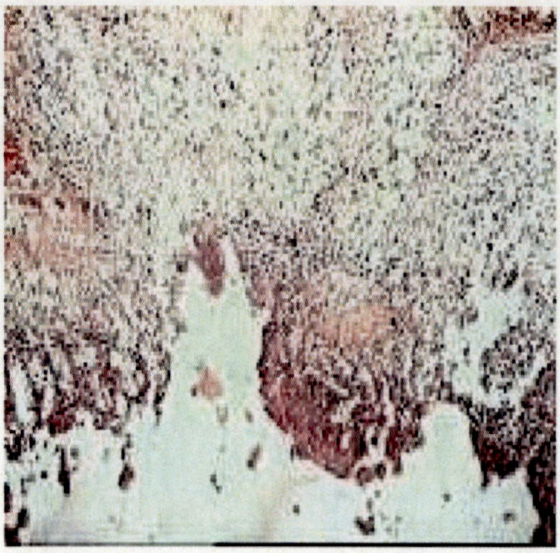

Fig.1.36: Photomicrograph of ulcer

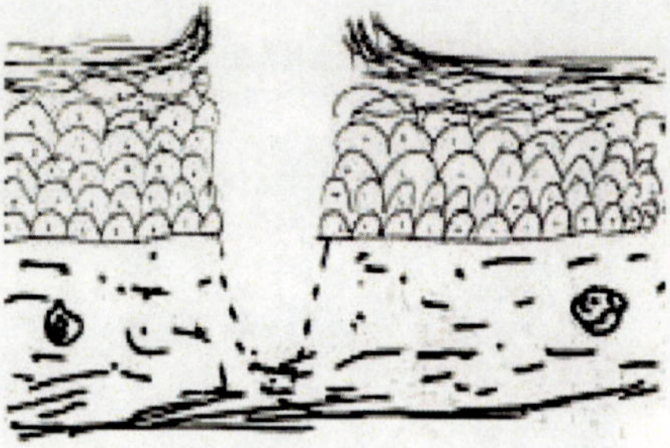

Fig. 1.37: Diagram of ulcer

Urticaria: A circumscribed area of swelling/ oedema involving dermis.

Folliculitis: Inflammation of hair follicles.

Acne: Enlargement of sealed off hair follicles or sebaceous glands and rupture through the epidermis. It leaves a rounded hole in the epidermis and a canal down to the dermis.

Eczema: Eczema is a form of allergic dermatitis of obscure etiology and characterized by erythema, vesicular rash, serous exudate and pruritus.

2

Pathology of Musculoskeletal System

Pathology of Muscles

Equine Rhabdomyolysis

It is also known as Azoturia or Monday Morning Disease. The disease occurs in well fed horse after a spell of inactivity. Suddenly after walking a few steps, the horse is unable to move further and feels pain with intense sweating and hardening of muscles.

Etiology

- Accumulation of lactic acid in muscles.
- High glycogen storage.
- Lack of oxygen supply.

Macroscopic features

- Hardening of muscle just like wood.
- Urine is dark brown with myoglobin – myoglobinuria.
- Tonic spasms in muscles.
- Atrophy of affected muscles in chronic cases.

Microscopic features

- Necrosis of muscle fibers
- Oedema.
- Hyaline degeneration (Fig. 2.1).

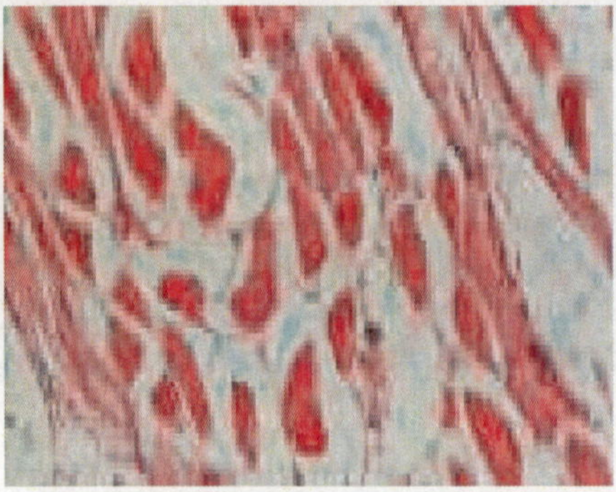

Fig. 2.1: Photomicrograph showing hyaline degeneration in muscle

- Invasion of sarcolemma by macrophages and lymphocytes.
- Degeneration and necrosis of tubular epithelium in kidneys.

White Muscle Disease

Extensive coagulative necrosis of muscles is observed in calves possibly due to deficiency of vitamin E during 6 months of age (Fig. 2.2).

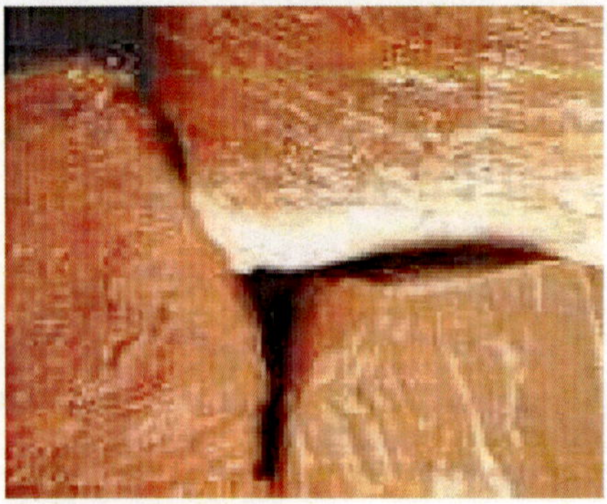

Fig. 2.2: Photograph of white muscle disease

Etiology

- Vitamin E deficiency.
- Selenium deficiency.
- Stress.

Macroscopic features

- Colour of muscle becomes pale pink, yellowish red, grey or white (Fig.2.3).

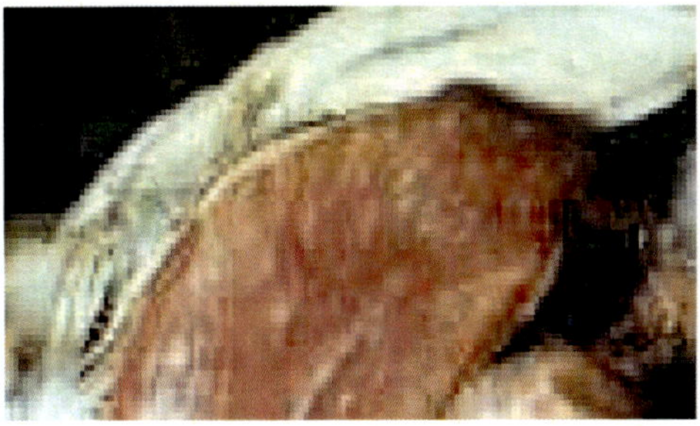

Fig. 2.3: Photograph showing muscular dystrophy

- Muscle becomes dry, inelastic and firm.
- Urine is brown/red or chocolate brown in colour because of myoglobin.

Microscopic features

- Coagulative necrosis of muscles.
- In some muscle cells, cloudy swelling can be observed.
- Neutrophils, macrophages, lymphocytes and eosinophils may be present.
- Calcium may be deposited in necrosed areas.

Acute Myositis

Acute myositis is the acute inflammation of skeletal muscles characterized by the presence of serous, fibrinous or hemorrhagic exudate (Figs. 2.4 & 2.5).

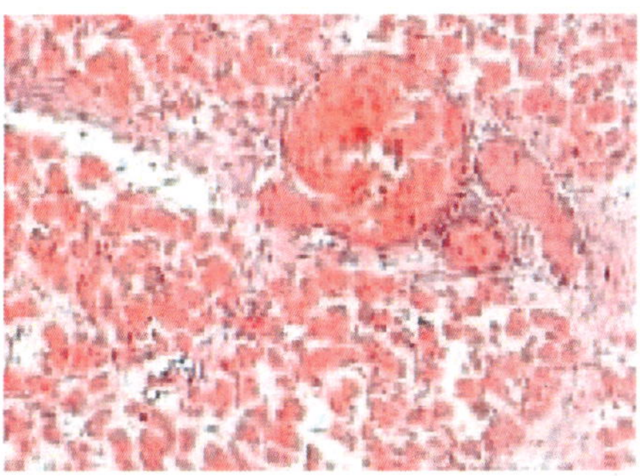

Fig. 2.4: Photomicrograph showing acute myositis

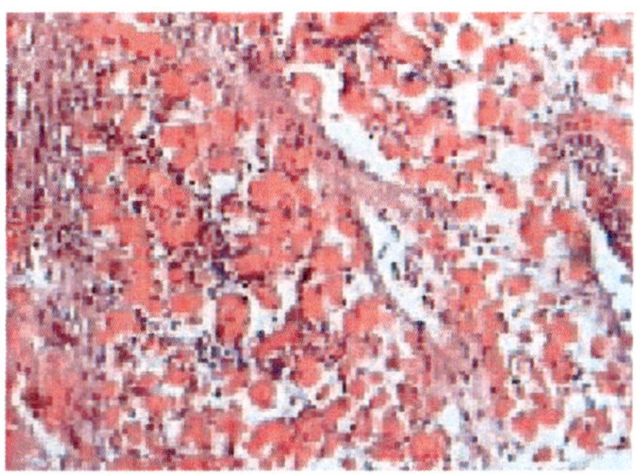

Fig. 2.5: Photomicrograph showing acute myositis due to *Clostridia* spp

Etiology

- Trauma.
- Vitamin E/Selenium deficiency.
- *Clostridium chauvei*, the cause of black leg in cattle.

Macroscopic features

- Muscles become extremely moist.
- Colour becomes red, consistency is firm and tense.
- Swelling and accumulation of gas in muscles, crepitating sound on palpation.
- Muscle dark red/ black with gas mixed exudate (Figs. 2.6 & 2.7) (gangrenous myositis).

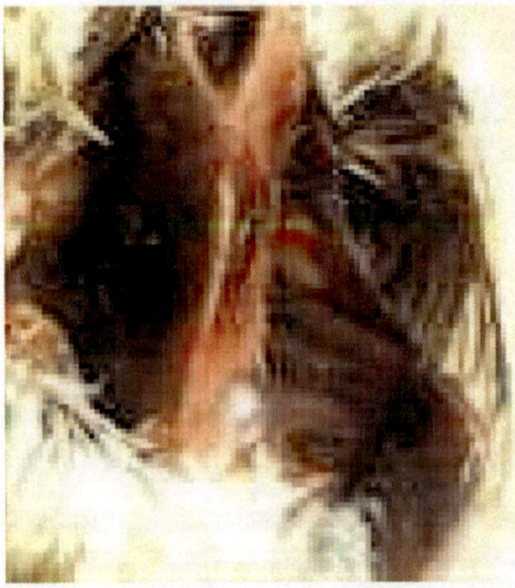

Fig. 2.6: Photograph showing gangrenous myositis in poultry

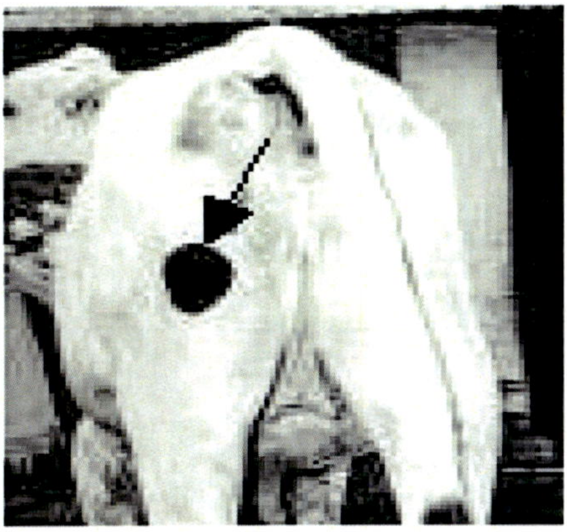

Fig. 2.7: Photograph showing gangrenous myositis in heifer

Microscopic features

- Presence of serous, fibrinous and/or hemorrhagic exudate.
- Infiltration of neutrophils, macrophages, lymphocytes, etc.
- Degenerative and necrotic changes in muscles.
- Presence of Gram positive rods in exudate.

Hemorrhagic Myositis

Hemorrhagic myositis is characterized by the presence of large amount of blood and inflammation in muscles. It may occur due to trauma and muscle rupture (Fig. 2.8).

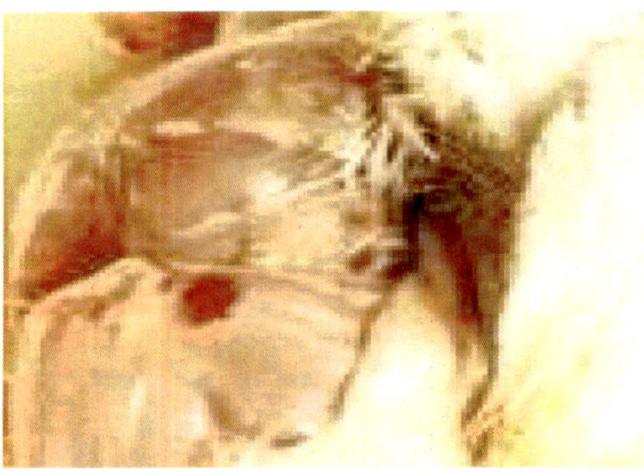

Fig. 2.8: Photograph showing hemorrhagic myositis

Etiology

- Trauma.
- Clostridial infections.

Macroscopic features

- Area becomes red/cyanotic.
- On cut, large amount of blood comes out from muscles.
- The affected area is hard and painful to touch.
- Regional lymphnodes may become enlarged and swollen.

Microscopic features

- Extravasation of blood in between the myofibrils.
- Infiltration of neutrophils, macrophages and lymphocytes in connective tissue between the muscle cells.

Chronic Myositis

Chronic inflammation of muscle is characterized by necrosis, calcification and proliferation of fibrous connective tissue. In case of tuberculosis and pseudotuberculosis, there are multiple focal nodules containing caseation and fibrous capsule.

Etiology

- Mycobacterium tuberculosis.
- Corynebacterium pseudotuberculosis.
- *Trichinella* spp. infection.
- *Sarcosporidia* spp. infection.

Macroscopic features

- Muscles become hard to touch.
- Nodules can be seen (Fig. 2.9).

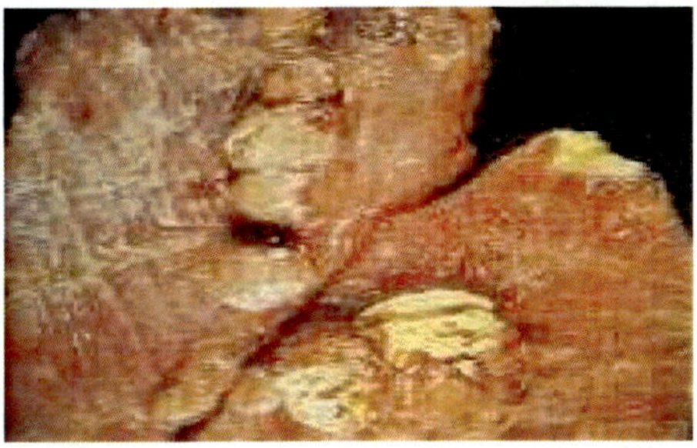

Fig. 2.9: Photograph showing chronic myositis

- On cut the lesions of caseation and calcification observed.

Microscopic features

- Caseative necrosis, infiltration of macrophages, lymphocytes and proliferation of fibrous tissue.
- Calcification can also be observed.
- In cases of pseudotuberculosis infiltration of neutrophils is seen.
- Extensive infiltration of eosinophils in sarcoporidia infection.

Pathology of Bones

Fibrous Osteodystrophy

Fibrous osteodystrophy occurs as excessive action of parathyroid hormone on bones and characterized by bone resorption with replacement by fibrous tissue, increased osteoid formation which does not get sufficient minerals for deposition and formation of cysts.

Etiology

- Hyperparathyroidism
- Dietary deficiency of calcium or excess of phosphorus
- Vitamin-D deficiency
- Excessive bran feeding (Disease in horses of flour millers).

Macroscopic features

- Lack of calcification in bone
- Resorption of calcium from bone, fibrosis

- Bone becomes soft, flexible and deformed
- Rubbery jaw due to involvement of facial bones

Microscopic features

- Fibrous tissue hyperplasia in bones.
- Enlargement of Haversian canals.
- Boney tissue is replaced by fibroblasts, with osteoclastic giant cells lining the remaining bone tissue.

Rickets

Rickets is failure of adequate deposition of calcium in bones of growing animals caused by deficiency of calcium and vitamin D and is characterized by bending of limbs, enlargement of ends of long bones and skeletal deformities (Fig. 2.10).

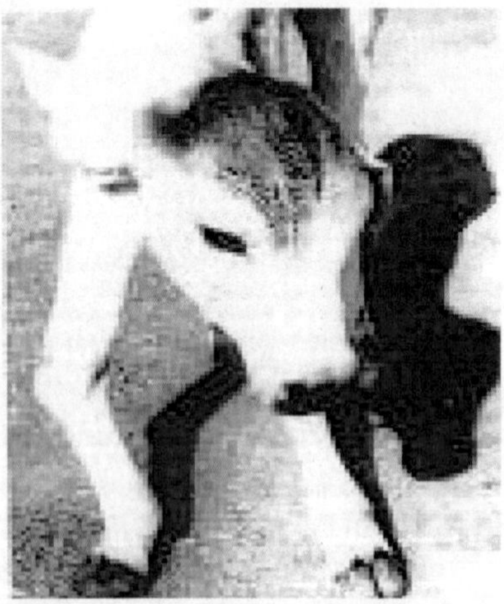

Fig. 2.10: Photograph of calf showing rickets

Etiology

- Vitamin D deficiency.
- Calcium deficiency.
- Deficiency of phosphorus.

Macroscopic features

- Bending of legs, bow legs.

- Pot belly.
- Enlarged costochondral articulation.
- Softening of bones.

Microscopic features

- Increase in proliferating cartilage adjacent to the area of ossification and its disorderly arrangement.
- Disorderly penetration of cartilage by blood vessels.
- Increased area of uncalcified osteoid tissue
- Fibrosis of marrow.

Osteomalacia

Osteomalacia is also known as adult rickets. It occurs in bone of adults and is caused by deficiency of vitamin D and calcium and characterized by softening of bones.

Etiology

- Vitamin D deficiency.
- Calcium-phosphorus ratio disturbance.

Macroscopic features

- Softening of bones.
- Irregular diffuse thickening of bones.
- Bone deformities.

Microscopic features

- Increase in osteoid tissue with failure of calcification.
- Increase in osteoclastic activity.

Osteoporosis

Osteoporosis is atrophy of bones caused by possibly hormonal imbalance and is characterized by inadequate deposition of calcium, brittleness of bones due to its increased porosity.

Etiology

- Hormonal imbalance.
- Vitamin C deficiency.
- Copper deficiency.

Macroscopic features

- Inadequate calcium deposition.
- Bone becomes brittle and porous.
- Increased fragility of bones.

Microscopic features

- Widening of Haversian canals.
- Increased activity of osteoclasts.
- Decrease in zona compacta and thickness of bone trabeculae.

Osteopetrosis

Osteopetrosis is enlargement of bone caused by fluorosis or avian leukosis virus and is characterized by increase in bony tissue. It is also known as marble bone disease.

Etiology

- Avian leukosis virus of retroviridae family.
- Fluorosis.

Macroscopic features

- Enlargement of bone towards outside and inside.
- Reduced marrow cavity.
- Bone becomes brittle, marbelling of bones.

Microscopic features

- Cartilage is also calcified, surrounded by osteoid tissue.

Osteomyelitis

Osteomyelitis is the inflammation of bone with bone marrow caused by trauma and pyogenic bacteria and is characterized by destruction, replacement and excessive growth of new bone adjacent to the infected part (Fig. 2.11).

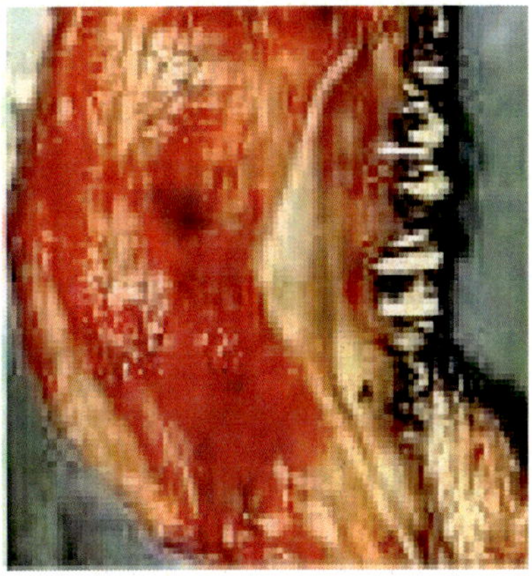

Fig. 2.11: Photograph showing osteomyelitis in mandible (Actinomycosis)

Etiology

- Hematogenous infection.
- Direct infection through trauma/fracture.
- *Actinomyces pyogenes, A. bovis.*
- *Staphylococcus aureus*.
- *Pseudomonas aeruginosa*.

Macroscopic features

- Metastatic abscess in bone marrow.
- Excessive growth of bone in adjacent area.
- Exostosis or endostosis.

Microscopic features

- Infiltration of neutrophils.
- Proliferation of osteoid tissue.
- Demonstration of bacteria in pus.

Bone Fracture and Repair

Fracture is the break in the continuity of bone due to trauma. A fracture may be simple or compound depending on the severity of trauma. Healing of fracture occurs by reunion of the broken ends of bone through development and proliferation of fibroblasts, angioblasts, osteoid tissue and infiltration of calcium salts (Figs. 2.12 & 2.13).

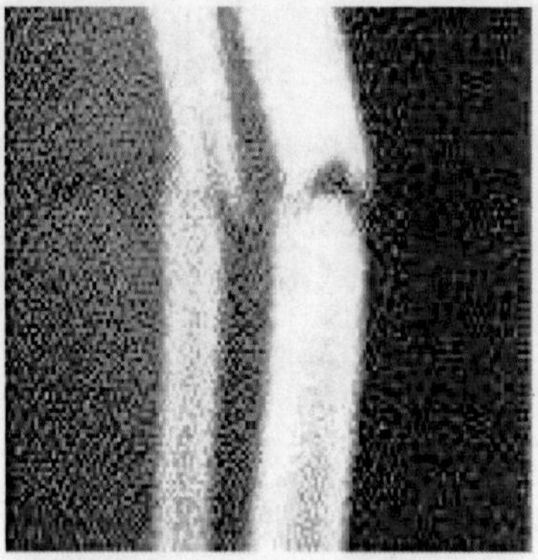

Fig. 2.12: Photograph showing fracture

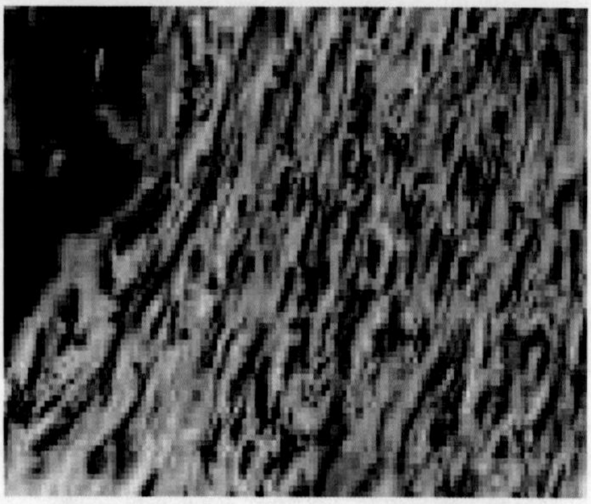

Fig. 2.13: Photomicrograph of fracture healing

Etiology

- Trauma.
- Accidents – automobile accidents.

Macroscopic features

- Fracture can be identified by break in bones.
- Healing of fracture is characterized by development of callus at the site of reunion of break ends of bone.
- Callus may be soft or hard.

Microscopic features

- Proliferation of fibroblasts, angioblasts and metaplasia of connective tissue to osteoid tissue.
- Areas of calcification in osteoid tissue

Pulmonary Osteoarthropathy

Pulmonary osteoarthropathy is a rare disease of dog, sheep, cat, horse, and lion caused by prolonged anoxia and is characterized by cough, dyspnea, respiratory disturbances and formation of new bone leading to thickening and deformity of limbs.

Etiology

- Prolonged anoxia.
- Toxaemia.

Macroscopic features

- Pneumonia.
- New bone formation due to hyperplasia just beneath the periosteum in long bones.
- The proliferation of bone is irregular leading to development of rough surface on bone.
- Bone becomes enlarged twice to its normal size.
- Heart worms were also seen in case of dogs.

Microscopic features

- Bronchogenic carcinoma.
- Granulomatous lesions of tuberculosis.
- Chronic bronchiectasis.
- Hyperplasia of osteoid tissue with no indication of any kind of neoplastic growth in bones.

Spondylitis

Spondylitis is the inflammation of vertebrae caused by bacteria/fungi and characterized by caseation, intraosseous abscess formation granulomatous lesions and fibrosis (Figs. 2.14 & 2.15).

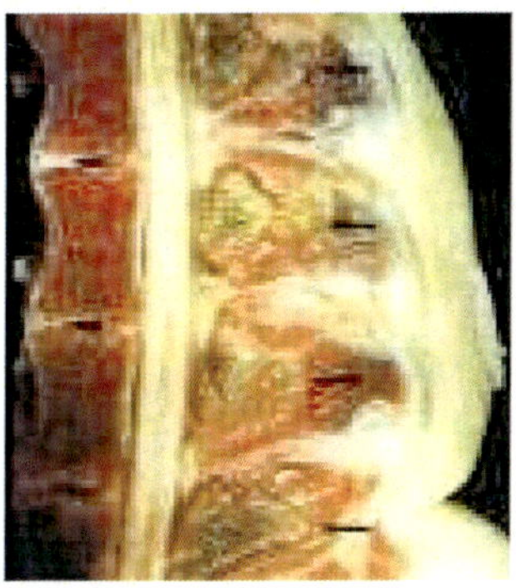

Fig. 2.14: Photograph showing spondylitis

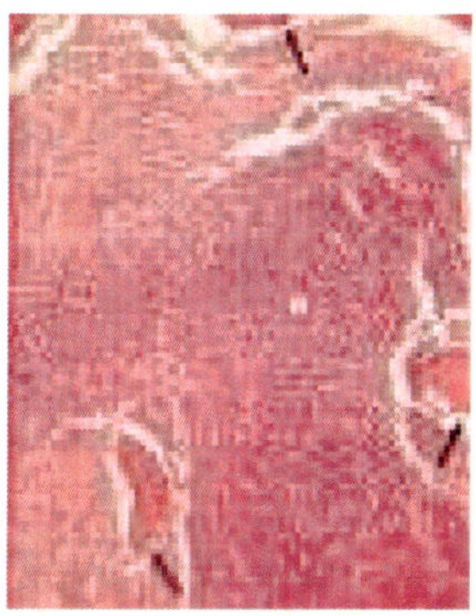

Fig. 2.15: Photomicrograph showing spondylitis

Etiology

- *Brucella abortus Br. Ovis, Br. Melitensis.*
- *Actinomyces bovis.*
- *Coccidioidomyces* sp.

Macroscopic features

- Intraosseous abscess.
- Granuloma encapsulated by fibrous tissue involving one or two adjacent vertebrae.
- Local enlargement of bone.

Microscopic features

- Granulomatous lesions with caseation.
- Proliferation of osteoid tissue.
- Infitration of neutrophils in intraosseous abscess.

Pathology of Joints

Arthritis

Arthritis is the inflammation of joint caused by bacteria, virus, chlamydia, mycoplasma and immune complexes and characterized by serus, fibrinous, purulent or ankylosing lesions in joints.

Etiology

- Bacteria – *E. coli*, *Erysipelas rhusiopathae*, *Streptococus* sp., *Shigella* sp. *Corynebacterium ovis*, *Brucella* sp.
- Mycoplasma – *Mycoplasma mycoides, Mycoplasma sinoviae*.
- Virus – Reovirus (Tenosynovitis in birds).
- Antigen antibody complexes.
- Trauma.

Macroscopic features

- Swelling of joints with increase in synovial fluid (Figs. 2.16 and 2.17).

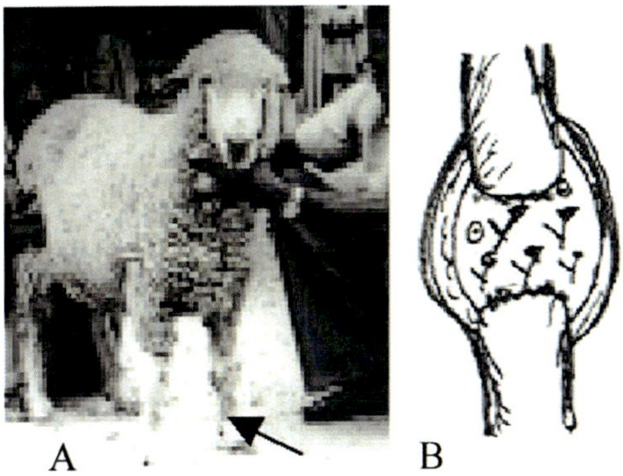

Fig. 2.16: A. Photograph showing arthritis
B. Diagram showing immune complex deposition in joint

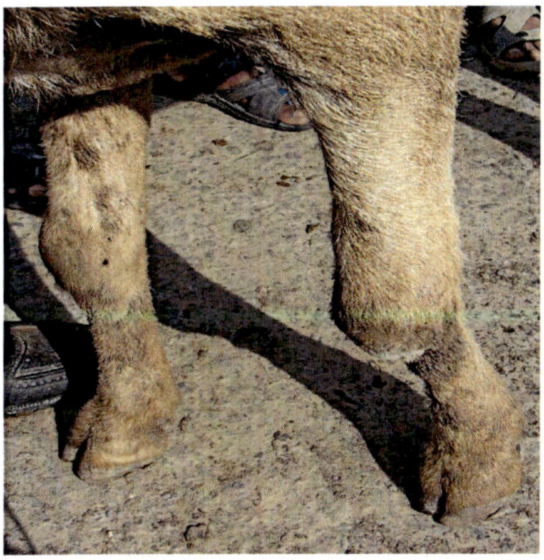

Fig. 2.17: Arthritis in cattle due to brucellosis.

- Difficulty in movement.
- In chronic cases fusion of two bony processes leaving no joint (ankylosing).
- Synovial fluid diminishes, becomes dirty, thick in chronic illness.

Microscopic features

- Presence of increased number of leucocytes in synovial fluid.
- Serous, fibrinous or purulent exudate in joints.
- Thickening of synovial membrane.
- Presence of plasma cells and immune complexes in synovial fluid.

3

Pathology of Cardiovascular System

Developmental Anomalies

Persistent right aortic arch

This is a developmental anomaly of aorta in which the aorta develops from right arch present on right side of trachea and oesophagus. The ductus arteriosus forms a ring around trachea and oesophagus by connecting aorta and pulmonary artery. This ring causes partial obstruction of trachea and/or oesophagus.

Patent ductus arteriosus

The ductus arteriosus is a short blood vessel which connects pulmonary artery to aorta in foetal life for diversion of blood. Normally, soon after birth this duct is sealed and remains in the form of a ligamentum arteriosum. But sometimes this ductus arteriosus remains open and blood is continuously shunted between aorta and pulmonary artery, after leading to congestive heart failure, pulmonary hypertension and cyanosis due to mixing of venous and arterial blood (Fig. 3.1).

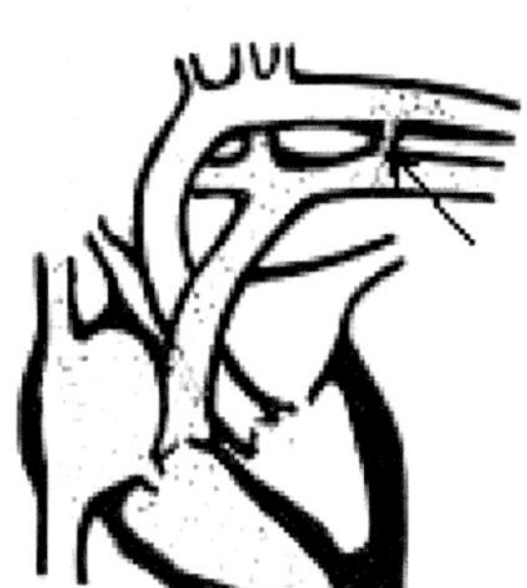

Fig. 3.1: Diagram of heart showing developmental anomaly patent ductus arteriosus

Interventricular septal defects

In foetal life, there is no partition in ventricles and there is only one chamber which is divided into two – right and left – by inter-ventricular septum. But when interventricular septum does not develop completely, or there is defect in formation of complete partition, there is mixing of blood from both chambers. It is responsible for thickening of myocardium, roughening of endocardium and cyanosis (Fig. 3.2).

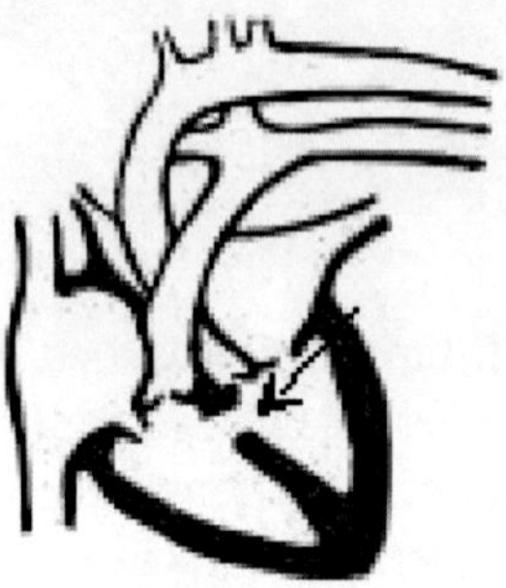

Fig. 3.2: Diagram of heart showing developmental anomaly interventricular septal defect

Transposition of aorta

This condition develops if there is a shift in position of aorta and pulmonary artery i.e. the aorta arises from right ventricle and pulmonary artery from left ventricle. This results in arterial blood in right and venous blood in left side and has no clinical significance. However, it may create problems when aorta arises from venous ventricle and pulmonary artery from arterial side.

Tetrad of Fallot

Tetrad of Fallot includes four developmental defects of cardiovascular system and is also known as tetralogy of Fallot (Fig. 3.3).

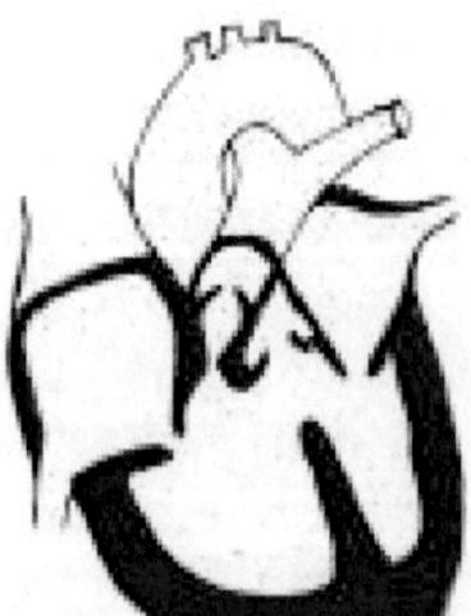

Fig. 3.3: Diagram of heart showing developmental anamalies tetralogy of fallot

1. Inter-ventricular septal defect.
2. Pulmonary stenosis is characterized by narrowing of lumen of pulmonary artery at its origin due to fibrous tissue causing 'jet' effect.
3. Hypertrophy of right ventricle.
4. Transposition of aorta.

Ectopia cordis

When heart lies outside the thorax under the subcutaneous tissue of lower cervical region.

Interatrial septal defect

There is a developmental defect in interatrial septa which remains as incomplete partition of atrium. It produces continuous overload on the right side of heart leading to pulmonary hypertension and hypertrophy of right side myocardium. However, a small defect in septum may persist throughout the life of animal without causing any clinical illness (Fig. 3.4).

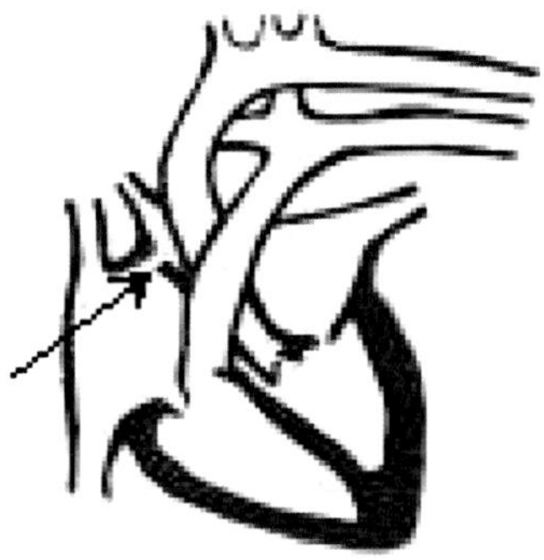

Fig. 3.4: Diagram of heart showing developmental anomaly interatrial septal defect

Cardiac Failure

Cardiac failure is the inability of heart to maintain adequate blood supply leading to death. It can be divided into two types: Acute and chronic heart failure.

Acute cardiac failure

Acute cardiac failure is sudden failure of contraction of heart leading to death within minutes.

Etiology

- Anoxia.
- Drugs/poisons.
- Shock.
- Cardiac temponade.
- Myocardial necrosis.
- Sudden occlusion of aorta and/or pulmonary artery.

Macroscopic features

- Cardiac temponade.
- Occlusive thrombus.
- Pulmonary congestion.
- Dilatation of heart particularly of right ventricle

Microscopic features

- Myocardial necrosis.
- Centrilobular necrosis in liver "***nut meg liver***".
- In prolonged cases, congestion and oedema in visceral organs.

Chronic Cardiac Failure

Chronic cardiac failure is the inability of heart to maintain balance between its output and venous return of blood. It can be further divided into two – left and right sided heart failure.

Left Sided Heart Failure

Left sided heart failure is caused by myocardial damage and is characterized by congestion and oedema in lungs with hypertrophy of alveolar lining cells (Fig. 3.5).

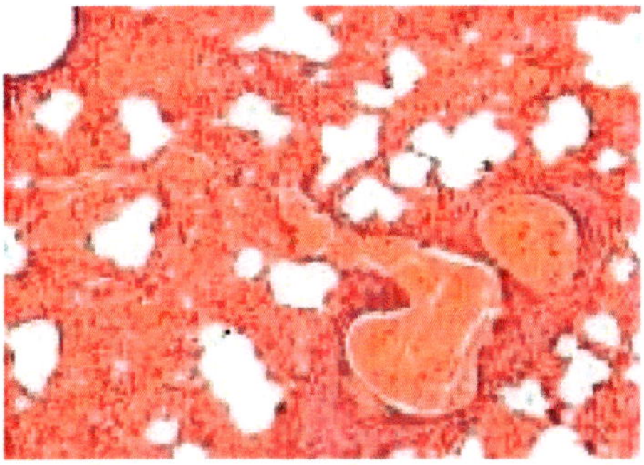

Fig. 3.5: Photomicrograph of lung showing lesions of heart failure

Etiology

- Myocardial degeneration/ necrosis
- Aortic and mitral valve disease
- Hypertension

Macroscopic features

- Congestion and oedema in lungs.
- Chronic dilatation of heart.

Microscopic features

- Congestion of alveolar vessels.
- Oedema in lungs.
- Hypertrophy of alveolar lining cells.
- Alveolar macrophages contain hemosiderin pigment also called "heart failure cells".

Right Sided Heart Failure

Right sided heart failure is caused by a disease of lungs or pulmonary vasculature and mostly occurs after a left sided heart failure.

Etiology

- Left sided heart failure.
- Pulmonary lesions, congestion.

Macroscopic features

- Congestion of visceral organs. Subcutis oedema and ascites.
- Pulse in jugular vein.

Microscopic features

- "Nutmeg appearance" in liver due to centrilobular necrosis.
- Atrophy, necrosis and fibrosis in liver.
- Congestion in visceral organs.

Pericarditis

Pericarditis is the inflammation of pericardium, the upper layer of heart. It may be serus, fibrinous or suppurative depending on the type of exudate.

Etiology/Occurrence

- Pasteurellosis.
- Salmonellosis in poultry (Fig. 3.6).

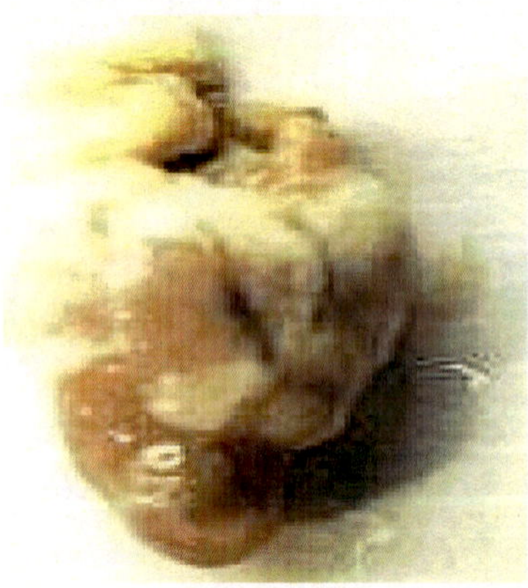

Fig. 3.6: Photograph of heart showing necrotic lesions due to *Salmonella Gallinarum* in poultry.

- Hydropericardium syndrome in poultry.
- Gout in poultry.
- Trauma/foreign body e.g. traumatic reticulo pericarditis (TRP) (Fig. 3.7).

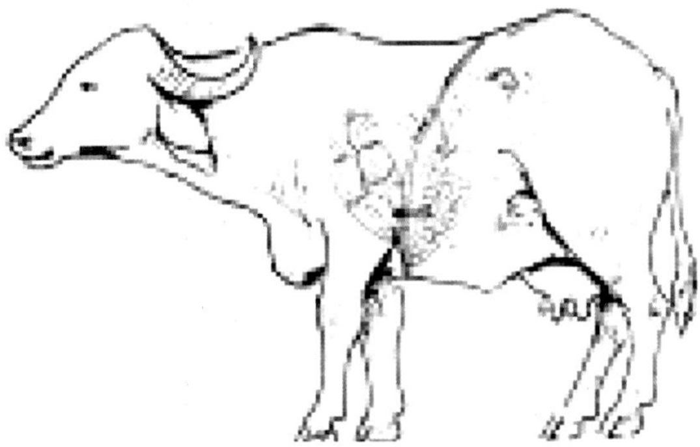

Fig. 3.7: Diagram showing traumatic reticulo pericarditis

Macroscopic features

- Deposition of fibrin in between pericardium and heart gives an appearance of "bread and butter" (Fig. 3.8).

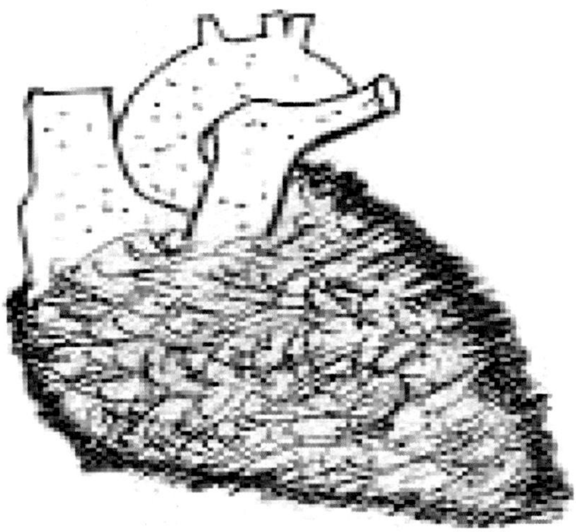

Fig. 3.8: Diagram showing fibrinous pericarditis

- In chronic cases, pericardium becomes thick due to excessive fibrosis.
- Accumulation of fluid (clear, serus) in pericardial sac is called Hydropericardium (Figs. 3.9 & 3.10).

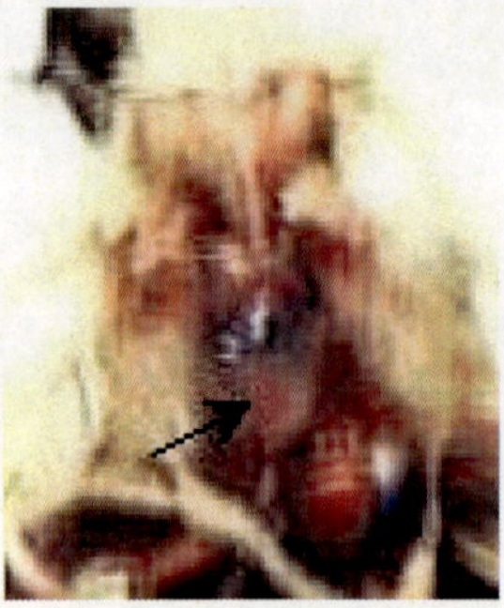

Fig. 3.9: Photograph of hydropericardium in poultry

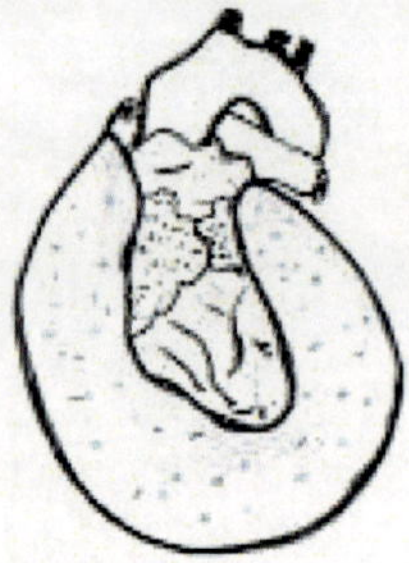

Fig. 3.10: Diagram showing hydropericardium

- Presence of blood in pericardial sac is known as hemopericardium and the excessive accumulation of blood leading to heart failure is termed as cardiac temponade (Fig. 3.11).

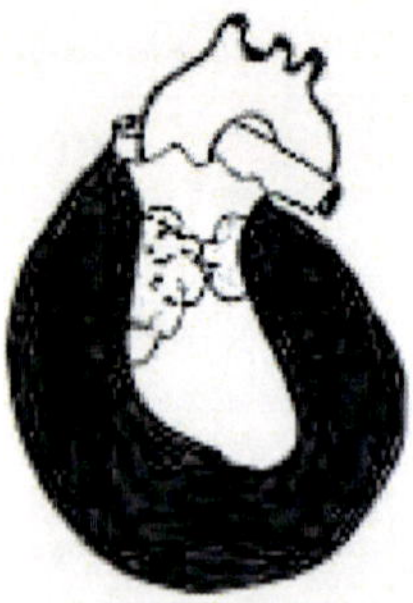

Fig. 3.11: Diagram showing hemopericardium (cardiac temponade)

- Accumulation of pus in pericardial sac is known as pyopericardium.
- Presence of gas in pericardial sac in known as pneumopericardium.

Microscopic features

- Hyperemia and hemorrhage in pericardium.
- Deposition of fibrin, formation of fibrin network, infiltration of neutrophils, macrophages and lymphocytes.

Myocarditis

Myocarditis is the inflammation of myocardium, the middle layer of heart. It may be suppurative, eosinophlic or lymphocytic depending on the type of the exudate (Figs. 3.12 & 3.13).

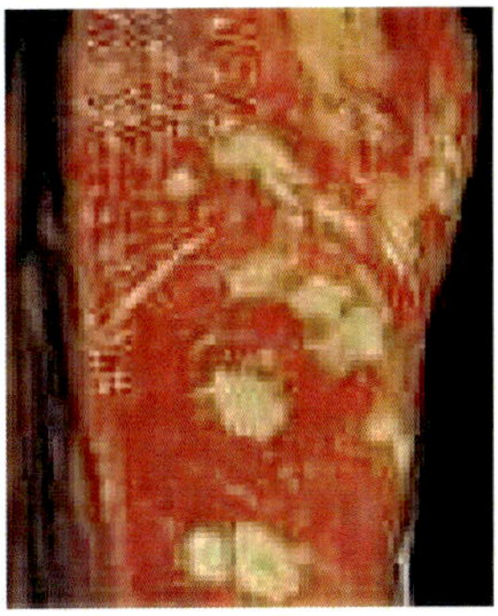

Fig. 3.12: Photograph showing myocarditis

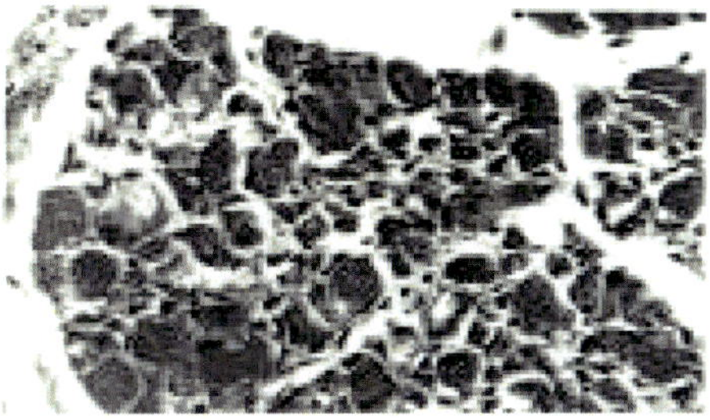

Fig. 3.13: Photomicrograph showing myocarditis

Etiology

- Toxins/ Poisons.
- Bacteria / Virus.
- Parasites.
- Drugs / Chemicals.

Macroscopic features

- Colour of myocardium may become dark red or cyanotic due to accumulation of blood.
- In suppurative myocarditis, one can find abscesses in myocardium from where yellow/ green pus oozes out.
- Yellowish white streaks of necrosis in myocardium.
- Presence of cyst encapsulated by fibroplasia due to cysticercosis.

Microscopic features

- Hyperemia and hemorrhage in myocardium.
- Infiltration of neutrophils, eosinophils or lymphocytes.
- Coagulative necrosis of muscle fibres.
- In chronic cases, proliferation of fibrous connective tissue.

Endocarditis

Endocarditis is the inflammation of the endocardium, the inner layer of heart (Figs. 3.14 to 3.20).

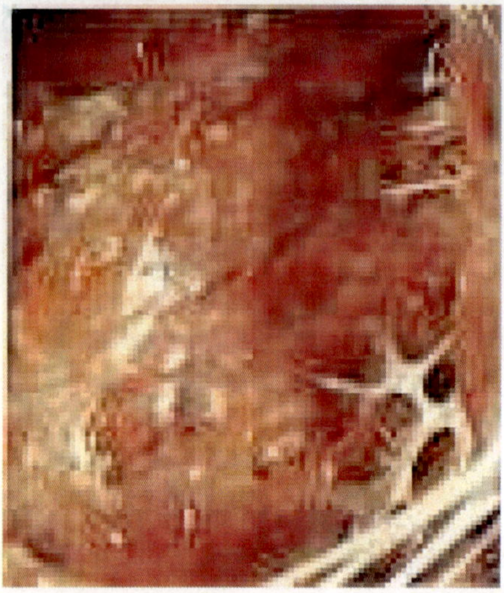

Fig. 3.14: Photograph showing endocarditis

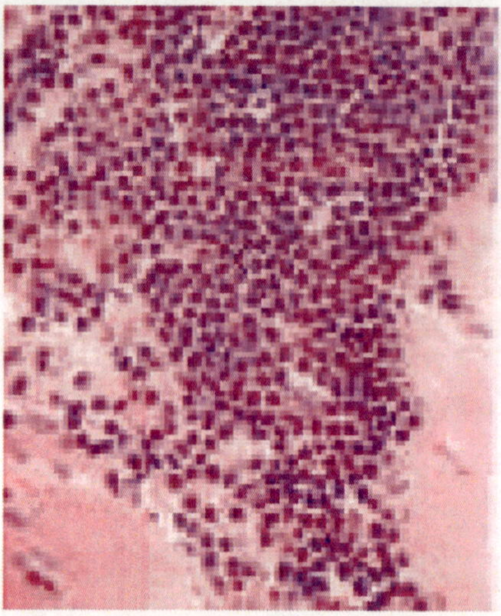

Fig. 3.15: Photomicrograph showing eosinophilic endocarditis

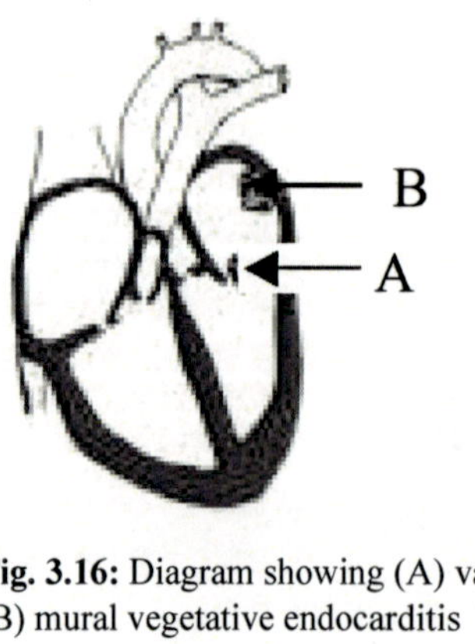

Fig. 3.16: Diagram showing (A) valvular and (B) mural vegetative endocarditis

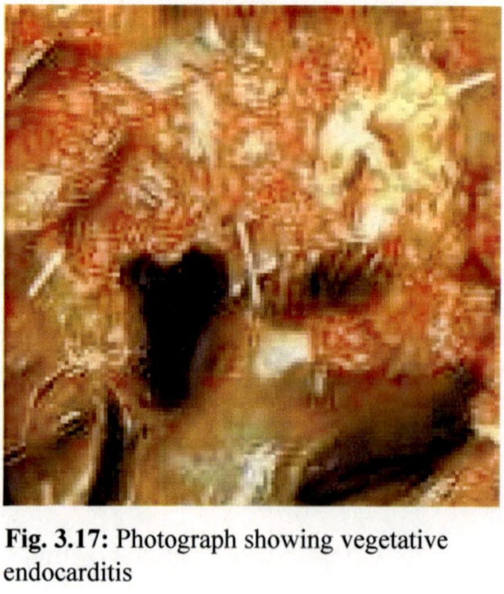

Fig. 3.17: Photograph showing vegetative endocarditis

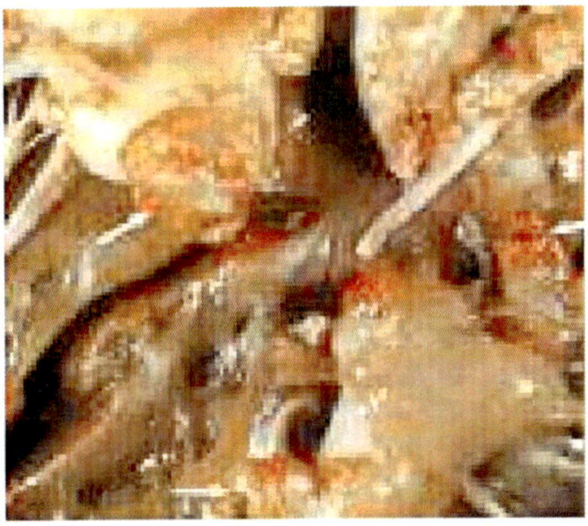

Fig. 3.18: Photograph showing vegetative endocarditis

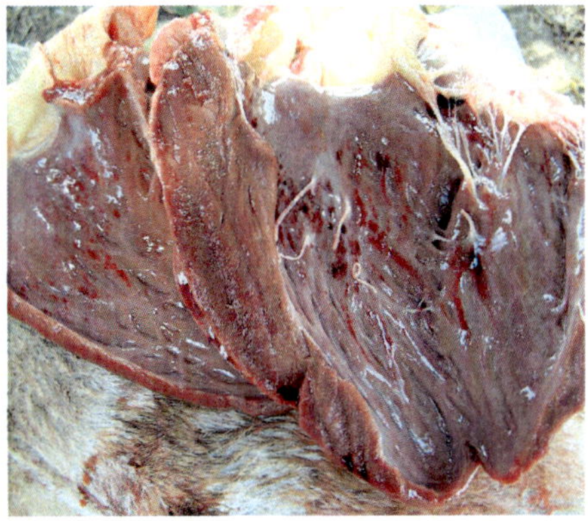

Fig. 3.19: Heart showing hemorrhagic endocarditis

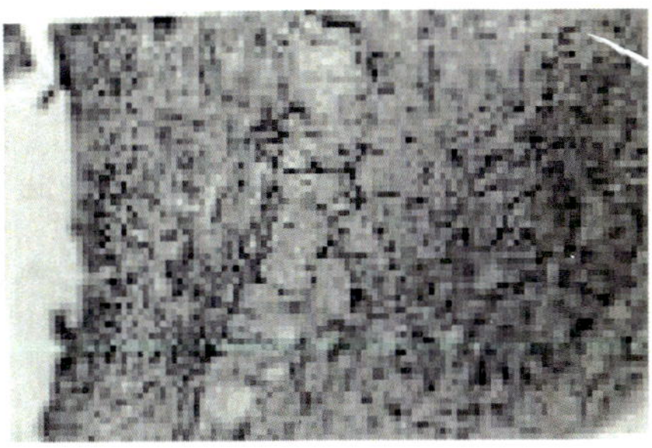

Fig. 3.20: Photomicrograph showing endocarditis

Etiology/ Occurrence

- Chronic septicemic diseases like caused by
  - *Actinomyces pyogenes*,
  - *Erysipelothrix rhusiopathiae*.
- Staphylococci.
- Streptococci.
- *Pseudomonas aeruginosa.*
- Clostridial infections.

Macroscopic features

- Lesions in heart valves or wall of atrium/ ventricles.
- Presence of thrombi on endocardium.

- Vegetative/cauliflower like growth on endocardium either in valves (Valvular vegetative endocarditis e.g. swine erysepalas) or in wall (Mural vegetative endocarditis).
- Dilation of heart chambers.

Microscopic features

- Infiltration of thrombocytes, neutrophils, macrophages and lymphocytes.
- Masses of bacterial organisms can be seen.
- Underlying endocardium and myocardium show the presence of fibrin network and infiltration of RBC, neutrophils and macrophages.

Brisket Disease / High Altitude Disease

Brisket disease is a condition of slow cardiac failure, which occurs at 2500 meters above sea level or higher where pressure of air is low (Fig. 3.21).

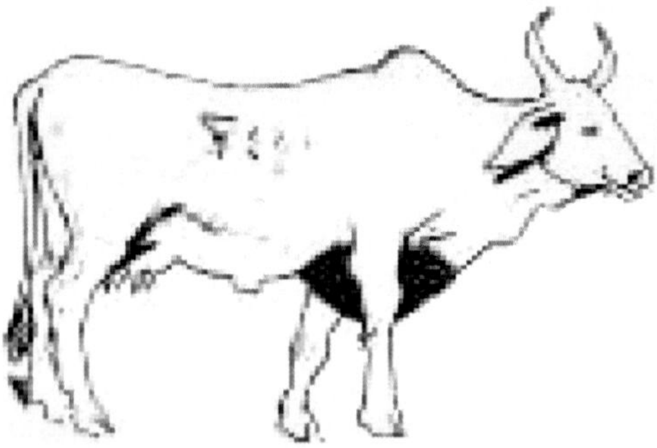

Fig. 3.21: Diagram showing Brisket disease in cow

Etiology

- Low oxygen in environment.
- Decreased atmospheric pressure of air.
- In native cattle morbidity rate is only 2% and in imported cattle at hills it is up to 40%.

Macroscopic feature

- Dilation of heart.
- Hypertrophy of ventricular wall.

- Chronic passive congestion in visceral organs.
- Oedema in sternal region in between forelegs.

Microscopic feature

- Nutmeg liver due to chronic passive congestion.
- Polycythemia.
- Hypertrophy of muscle fibers in myocardium.

Mulberry Heart Disease

It is characterized by firm contraction of heart and petechial hemorrhage on pericardium giving the appearance of mulberry.

Etiology

- Not known
- May be enterotoxaemia/poisoning

Macroscopic features

- Contraction of heart with petechial hemorrhage on pericardium looking like mulberry "***Mulbery heart disease***"
- Hydropericardium, hydroperitoneum and pulmonary oedema
- Oedema fluid has high protein content resulting in clot formation
- Congestion of fundic portion of stomach.

Microscopic features

- Congestion on serosa of visceral organs.

Arteriosclerosis

Arteriosclerosis is hardening of arteries causing 3 types of diseases in arteries depending on their size and etiological factors viz., Atherosclerosis, medial sclerosis and arteriolosclerosis.

Atherosclerosis

Atherosclerosis is characterized by hardening and thickening of intimal layer of large arteries and aorta due to proliferation of connective tissue, hyaline degeneration, infiltration of fat/ lipids and calcification. These intimal changes may lead to loss of elasticity of artery (Athere means mushy substance) (Fig. 3.22 & Fig. 3.23).

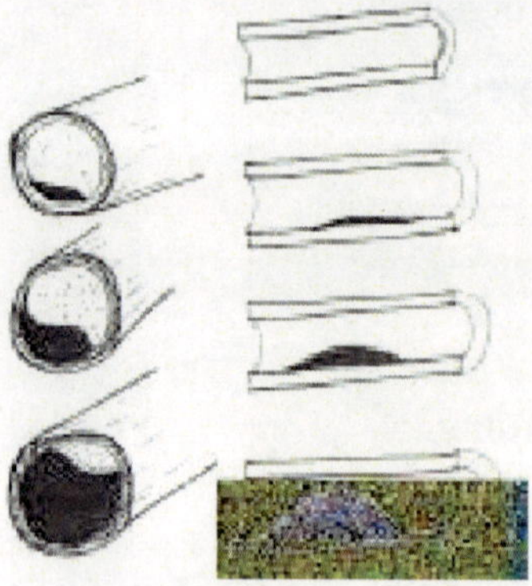

Fig. 3.22: Diagram showing atherosclerosis leading to obstruction of vessel

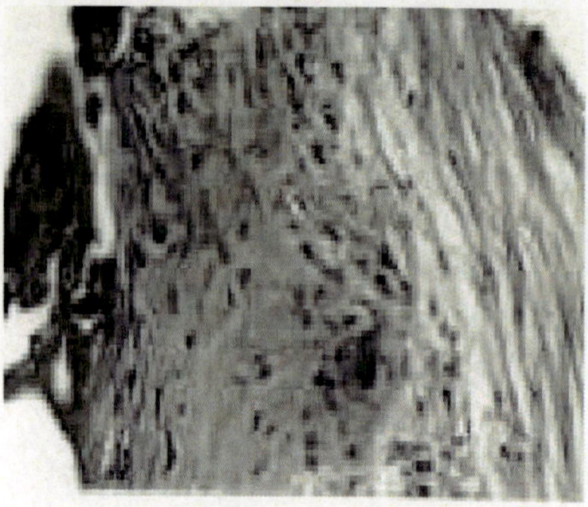

Fig. 3.23: Photomicrograph showing arteriosclerosis

Etiology

- Exact cause is not clear
- Hypercholesterolemia and hyperlipidemia
- Hypertension

Macroscopic features

- Fatty streaks running parallel in the direction of the artery.
- Intimal layer of aorta/ coronary arteries is elevated due to plaques which are white/ yellow, fibrous and occluding the lumen of vessel.
- Occlusion of artery may lead to ischemia and infarction.

Microscopic features

- Macrophages are filled with lipid droplets including cholesterol, fatty acids, triglycerides and phospholipids.
- Fragmented internal elastic lamina in the intimal layer of artery
- Proliferation of altered smooth muscles may become metaplastic to macrophages.
- Deposition of mucoid ground substance and collagen fibers
- Hyalinization of connective tissue "***Fibrous plaques***".
- Presence of some fat droplets in between the lesion

Medial Sclerosis

Medial sclerosis involves medium sized muscular arteries and characterized by fatty degeneration and hyalinization of muscular tissue of medial arteries leading to necrosis. This is also known as ***"Monckeberg medial sclerosis"***.

Etiology

- Old age.
- Excessive administration of epinephrine (adrenaline).
- Nicotine.
- Vitamin D toxicity.
- Hyperparathyroidism.

Macroscopic features

- Hardening of medium sized arteries.
- Hyaline, fatty changes and calcification of arterial wall.

Microscopic features

- Fatty changes, hyalinization of muscular layer of medium sized arteries.
- Necrosis of myofibrils.
- Calcification.

Arteriolosclerosis

Arteriolosclerosis affects arterioles in kidneys, spleen and pancreas and is characterized by hyperplasia of intimal cells of arterioles producing concentric lamellations occluding their lumen.

Etiology

- Hypertension.

Macroscopic features

- No characteristic macroscopic lesion.
- Atrophy of organ, hardening.

Microscopic features

- Proliferation of cells present in intima of blood vessels.

- Swelling and necrosis of cells in medial layer leading to occlusion of lumen.
- Calcification in chronic cases.

Arteritis

Arteritis is the inflammation of arteries characterized by infiltration of neutrophils, lymphocytes and macrophages in the media and intima of arterial wall (Figs. 3. 24 & 3.25).

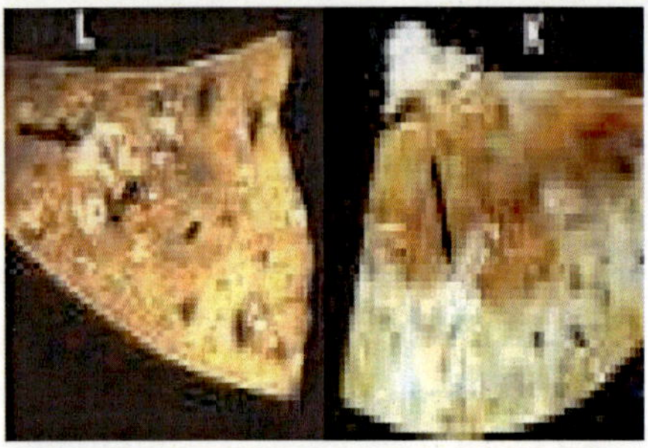

Fig. 3.24: Photograph showing arteritis (L) Liver (K) Kidney

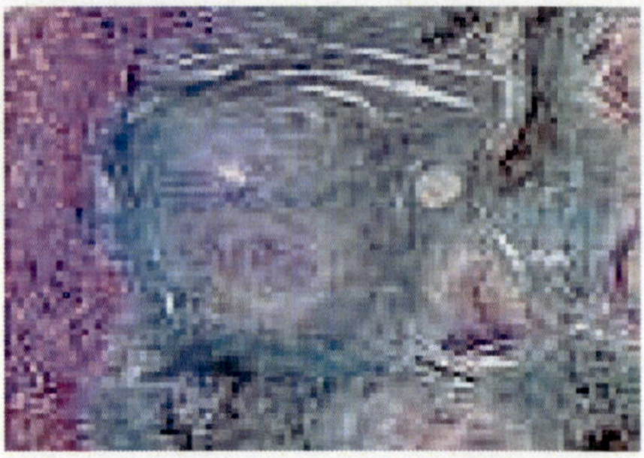

Fig. 3.25: Photomicrograph showing arteritis

Etiology

- Chemicals.
- Thermal.
- Virus e.g. Equine viral arteritis.
- Pyogenic bacteria.
- Parasite e.g. *Strongylus vulgaris*.

Macroscopic features

- Hyperemia.
- Conjunctivitis, oedema of eye.
- Presence of thrombi in artery.

Microscopic features

- Presence of thrombi in artery involving intimal layer.
- Equine viral arteritis virus causes infiltration of lymphocytes and macrophages in media.

- Occlusion of lumen of arteries due to thickening of wall.
- In parasitic arteritis, parasitic thrombi may present along with inflammatory reaction in intimal layer.

Aneurysm

Aneurysm is dilation of an artery or cardiac chamber leading to formation of sac (Fig. 3.26).

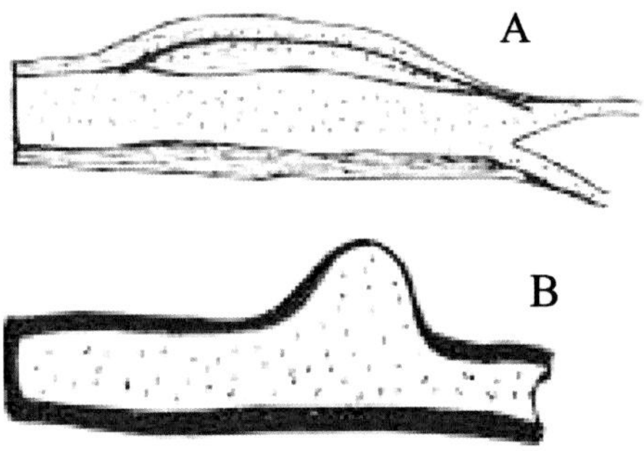

Fig. 3.26: Diagram showing aneurysm (a) dissecting (b) sacular

Etiology

- Aflatoxin.
- Infectious emboli.
- Weak vessel wall due to rupture.
- Fracture or necrosis of medial layer of large blood vessel.
- Arteriolosclerosis.

Macroscopic features

- Fracture or necrosis of medial layer of large blood vessels permitting parallel blood circulation till the next division of blood vessel is called as Dissecting aneurysm or false aneurysm.
- Formation of sac in artery due to dilation, also known as True aneurysm.

Microscopic features

- Rough intimal layer.
- Wall of blood vessel damaged with inflammatory exudate.

Phlebitis

Phlebitis is the inflammation of veins characterized by presence of inflammatory exudate, thickening of the wall and dilation of the lumen (Fig. 3.27).

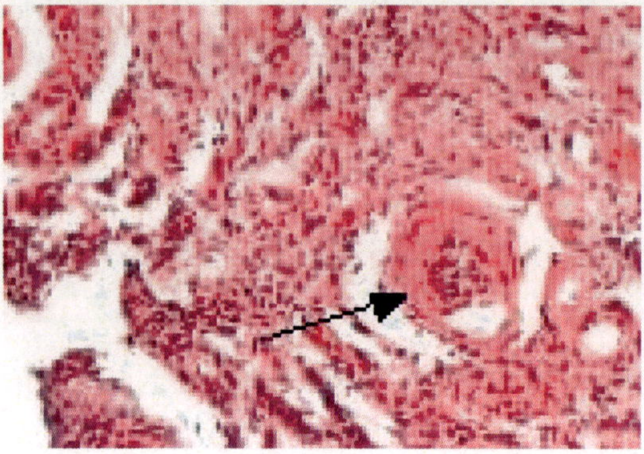

Fig. 3.27: Photomicrograph showing phlebitis

Etiology/Occurrence

- Naval infection in calves.
- Uterine infections
- In jugular vein due to improper intravenous infection.
- Varicose veins are dilated and elongated veins following irregular and tortuous course.
- Telangiectasis is marked dilation of veins particularly of sinusoidal capillaries in one or more lobules in liver.

Macroscopic feature

- Wall of vein is thickened.
- Vein contains large thick necrotic material
- Lumen dilated
- Inner surface of vein is rough and hyperemic.

Microscopic feature

- Infiltration of neutrophils in the wall of veins
- Sometimes calcification may also present.
- Wall of vein becomes thick due to inflammatory cells and/or proliferation of fibrous tissue.

Lymphangitis

Lymphangitis is the inflammation of lymph vessels characterized by aggregation of lymphocytes around lymphatics, oedema of dependent parts and distension of lymphatics (Fig. 3.28).

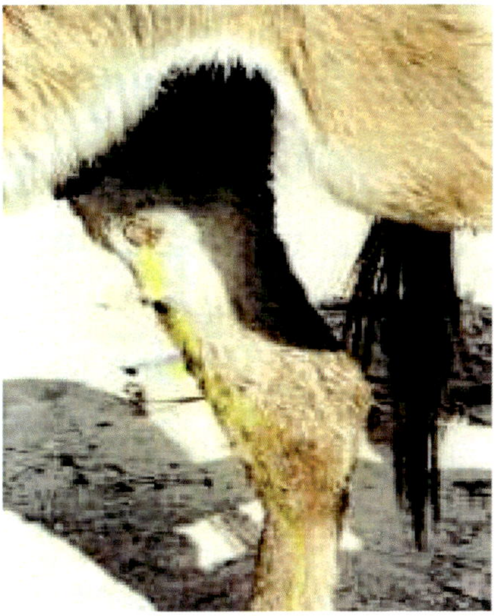

Fig. 3.28: Photograph showing of lymphangitis

Etiology/Occurrence

- *Corynebacterium ovis* causes caseous lymphangitis and lymphadenitis
- Equine epizootic lymphangitis

Macroscopic lesions

- Distension of subcutaneous lymph vessels, nodules of lymphoid aggregates.
- Oedema due to failure of lymphatic drainage.

Microscopic lesions

- Lymphoid aggregation around lymphatics.
- Lymphatics distended.
- Oedema of dependent tissue.

4

Pathology of Respiratory System

Pathology of Upper Respiratory Tract

In many infectious diseases, there is inflammation of mucosa of upper respiratory passage leading to nasal discharge which is catarrhal, purulent or fibrinous, depending on the type of infection. The infection may extend to lower parts of respiratory tract and reach the lungs causing pathological alterations. Rhinitis is the inflammation of nasal mucosa (Fig. 4.1). Sinusitis is the inflammation of sinuses e.g. frontal sinusitis in dehorned cattle. The larvae of botfly *Oestrus ovis* enter the nasal passage and migrate up to frontal sinuses and turbinate bones and cause mucopurulent inflammation. Similarly, leeches (*Dinobdella ferox*) is known to cause nasal cavity inflammation in domestic animals and suck blood. Rhinitis is caused by *Bordetella bronchiseptica* in pigs and is characterized by mucopurulent exudate, disappearance of nasal septum, retarded growth of snout and plugging of passage by solidified exudate and dead tissue. This condition is known as porcine atrophic rhinitis. Epistaxis is bleeding from nasal passage due to trauma, neoplasm (Fig.4.2A) and ulcerative lesions as a result of infections (Fig.4.2B). Pharyngitis is the inflammation of pharynx while laryngitis is the inflammation of larynx.

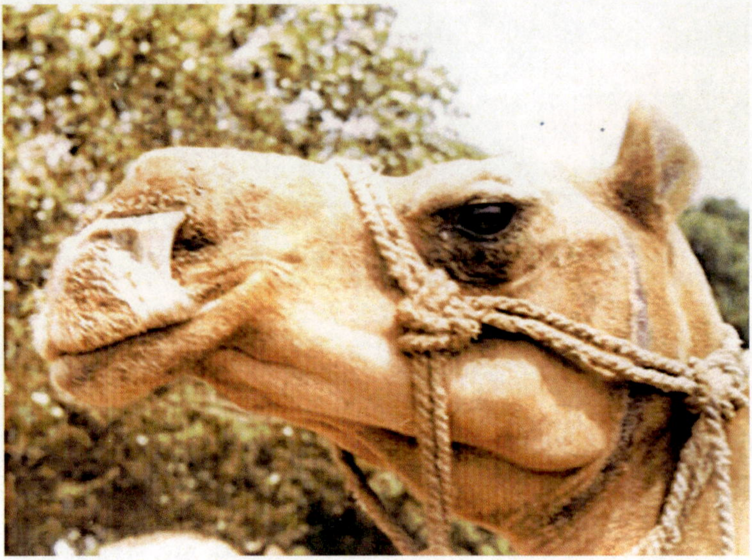

Fig. 4.1: Photograph showing rhinitis in a camel and catarrhal nasal discharge

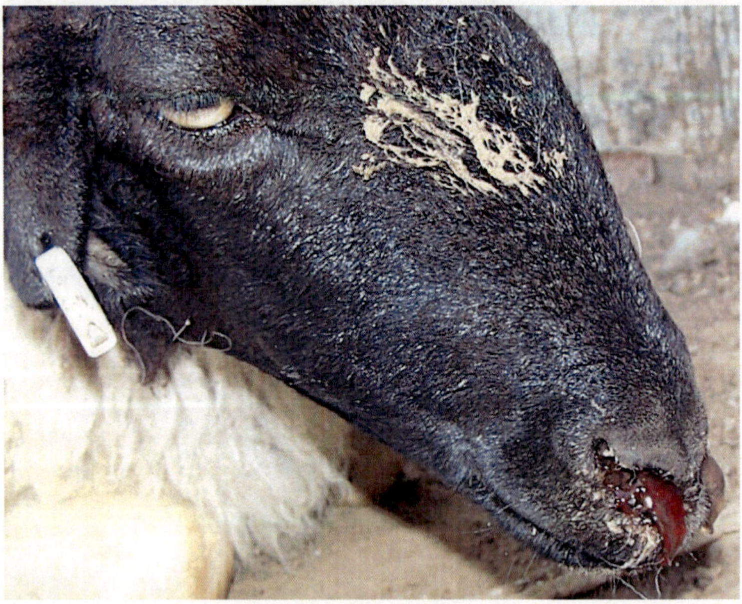

Fig. 4.2A: Photograph showing epistaxis in a sheep

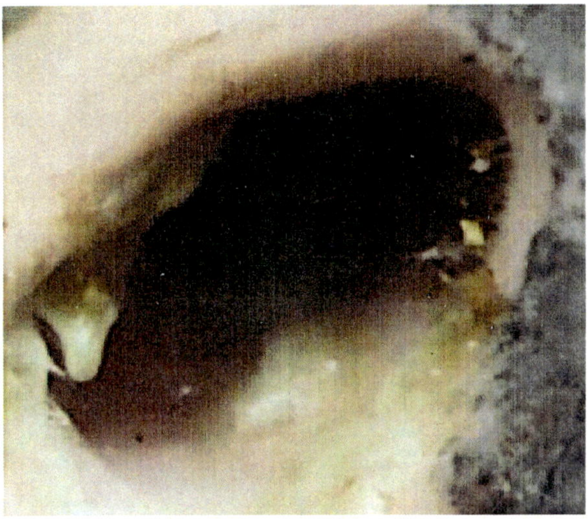

Fig. 4.2B: Ulcer and thick suppurative exudate in external nares.

Nasal Polyps

Nasal polyps are the inflammatory conditions of respiratory mucosa resembling neoplastic growth caused by fungus and characterized by formation of new growth simulating benign neoplasm in nasal passage.

Etiology

- *Rhinosporidium sceberi*, a fungus most commonly prevalent in southern India.

Macroscopic features

- Formation of a single polyp in respiratory mucosa, pedunculated, elongated, fills nasal cavity.
- Cauliflower like growth may cause bleeding.

Microscopic features

- Fibrous covering by mucous membrane and heavily infiltrated by neutrophils, lymphocytes, eosinophils, macrophages around fungus.

Nasal Granuloma

Nasal granuloma is the granulomatus inflammation of respiratory mucosa in nasal cavity caused by blood flukes and characterized by the presence of granulomatous growth filling the nasal passage causing obstruction (Figs. 4.3 & 4.4).

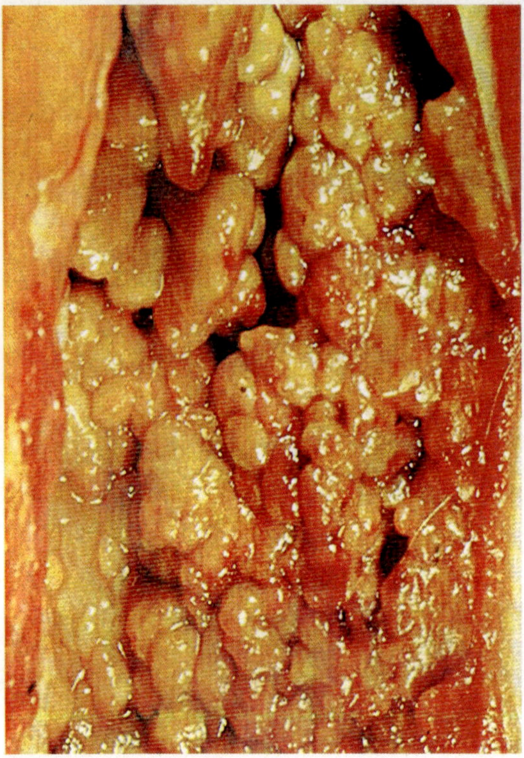

Fig. 4.3: Photograph showing nasal granuloma

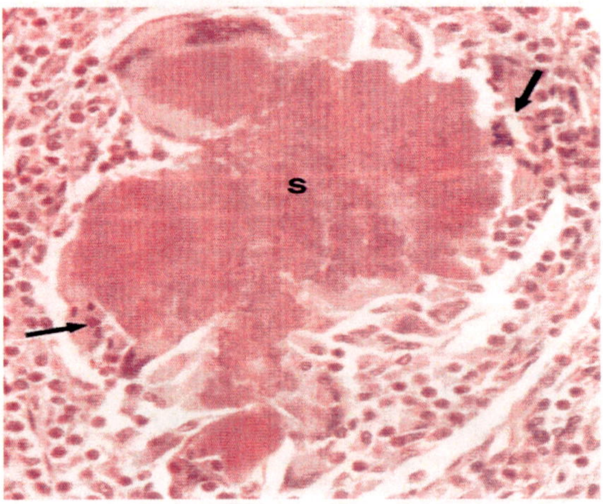

Fig. 4.4: Photomicrograph showing nasal granuloma

Etiology

- *Schistosoma nasalis*, a blood fluke.
- Type II hypersensitivity reaction of nasal mucosa to plant pollens, fungi, mites etc (Fig. 4.5).

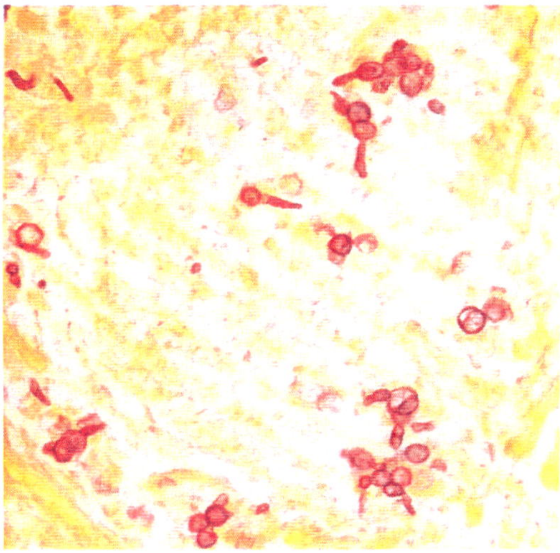

Fig. 4.5: Photomicrograph showing causative fungus in nasal granuloma

Macroscopic Features

- Nasal pruritus.
- Small tiny nodules on nasal mucosa later becomes cauliflower-like growth filling the cavity and causing obstruction.

Microscopic features

- Oedema in lamina propria.
- Infiltration of eosinophils, mast cells, lymphocytes and plasma cells and absence of epithelioid cells.
- Proliferation of fibroblasts.
- The lesion is covered by squamous epithelium.
- Mucous glands may have metaplastic pseudostratified columnar epithelium.

Tracheitis

Tracheitis is the inflammation of trachea. In canines, it is tracheobronchitis while in poultry it is manifested by laryngotracheitis (Fig. 4.6).

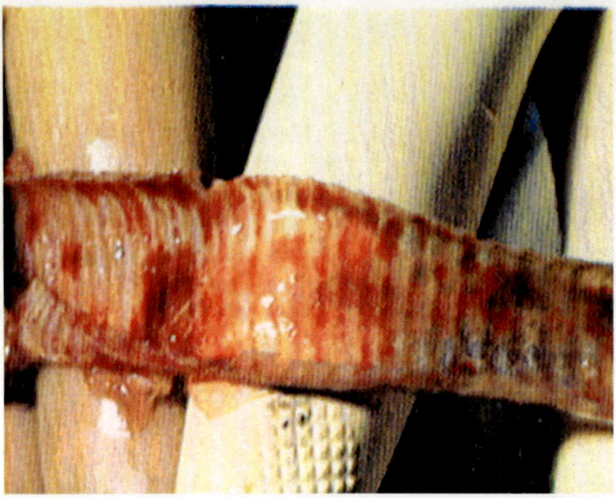

Fig. 4.6: Photograph showing haemorrhagic tracheitis in poultry

Etiology

- Canine tracheobronchitis caused by adenovirus, influenza virus and herpes virus.
- Avian infectious laryngotracheitis (ILT) is caused by herpes virus.

Macroscopic features

- Canine tracheobronchitis or kennel cough includes congestion of trachea and presence of catarrhal exudate.
- In poultry, hemorrhage in trachea and caseous plug in trachea towards larynx causing obstruction (Figs. 4.7 & 4.8).

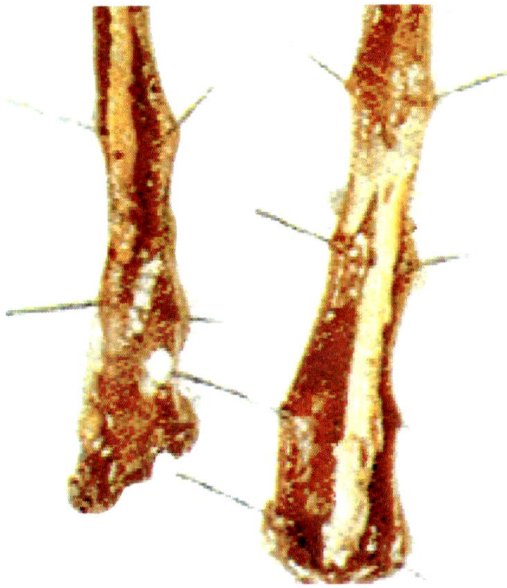

Fig. 4.7: Photograph showing presence of caseous exudate in larynx and trachea.

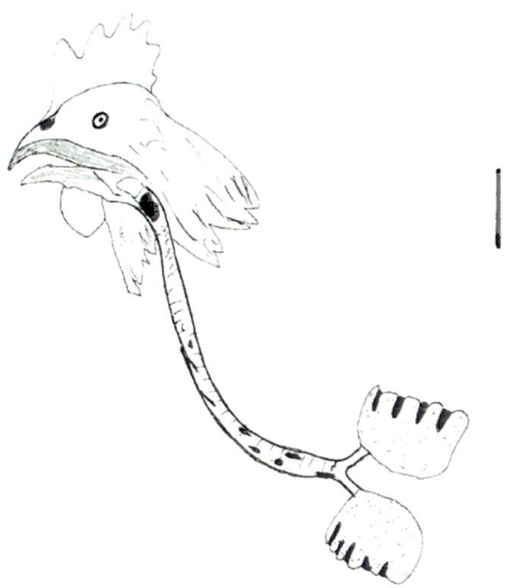

Fig. 4.8: Diagram showing presence of caseous exudates in larynx and trachea.

Microscopic features

- Inclusion bodies in tracheal and bronchial epithelium in canines.
- Hemorrhagic tracheitis, presence of intra nuclear basophilic inclusions in tracheal epithelial cells in infectious laryngotracheitis.

Bronchitis

Bronchitis is the inflammation of bronchi, characterized by catarrhal, suppurative, fibrinous or hemorrhagic exudate.

Etiology

- Bacteria e.g. Pasteurella.
- Virus e.g. infectious bronchitis in poultry.
- Parasites.
- Allergy/ Inhalation of pollens etc.

Macroscopic features

- Coughing, dyspnoea.
- Mucous exudate in lumen.
- Congestion and/or hemorrhages in bronchi.
- Presence of caseous plugs at the point where bronchi enter in lungs in infectious bronchitis of poultry (Fig. 4.9).

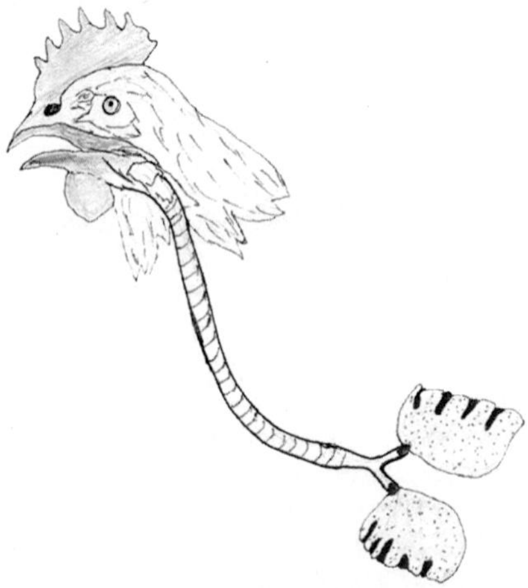

Fig. 4.9: Diagram showing lesions of infectious bronchitis in poultry

Microscopic features

- Mucous exudate along with inflammatory cells in the lumen of bronchi.
- Hyperplasia and/or necrosis of bronchiolar epithelium.
- Accumulation of mononuclear cells in the bronchial mucosa and in area.

Pathology of Lungs

Atelectasis

Atelectasis is the failure of alveoli to open or the alveoli are collapsed and thus do not have air.

Etiology

- Obstruction in bronchi/ bronchiole.
- Pleuritis.
- Atelectasis neonatorum in new born animals. In the absence of respiration, lung alveoli remain closed and thus sink in water indicating still birth.

Macroscopic features

- Dull red in colour, hard area of lung like liver in consistency.
- Atelectic lung sinks in water.

Microscopic features

- Compressed alveoli (Fig. 4.10).
- Absence of air spaces.
- Collapsed bronchioles.
- In inflammatory condition, exudate compresses alveoli.

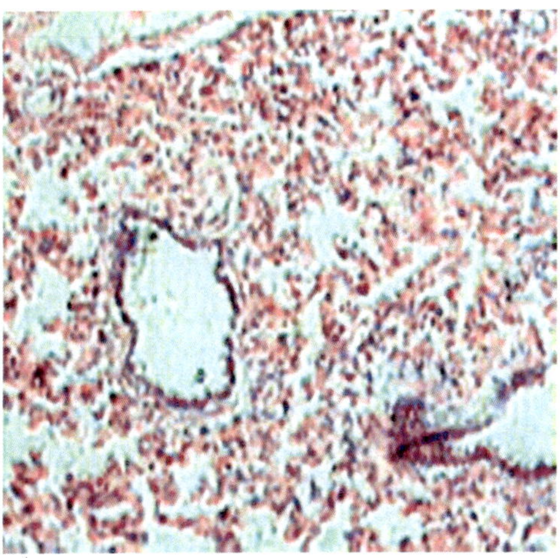

Fig. 4.10. Photomicrograph of lung showing atelectasis.

Emphysema

Emphysema is the increase in amount of air in lungs characterized by dilation of the alveoli. It may be acute or chronic and focal or generalized.

Etiology

- Bronchitis.
- Atelectasis in adjoining area of lung.
- Pneumonia.
- Allergy to dust, pollens etc.
- Pulmonary adenomatosis.

Macroscopic features

- Lungs are enlarged and flabby.
- Imprints of ribs can be seen. Colour of lungs becomes pale.
- Cut surface is smooth and dry.

Microscopic features

- Alveoli are distended (Fig. 4.11).

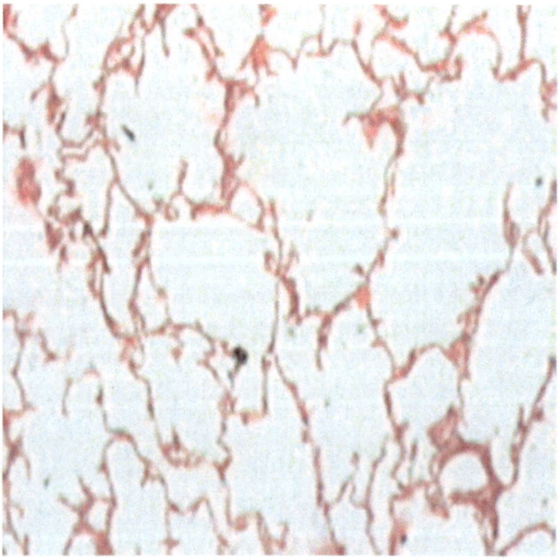

Fig. 4.11: Photomicrograph of lung showing emphysema

- Some alveoli may rupture and form giant alveoli.
- Alveolar wall becomes thin due to stretching.
- Mild bronchitis.
- Hyperplasia of lymphoid tissue.

Pulmonary Oedema

In pulmonary oedema, there is accumulation of serous fluid in alveoli of lungs (Figs. 4.12 & 4.13).

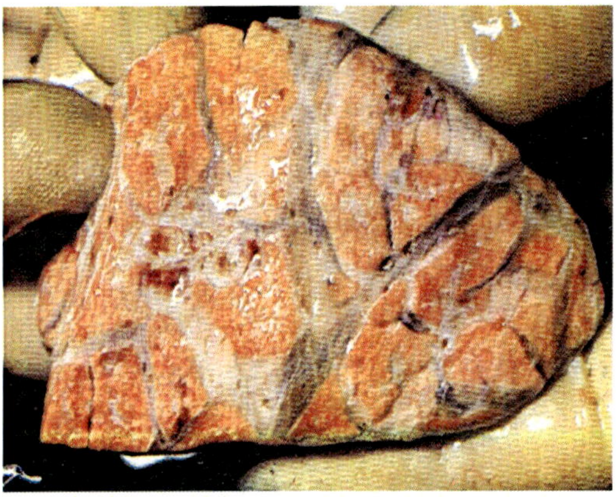

Fig. 4.12: Photograph of lung showing odema

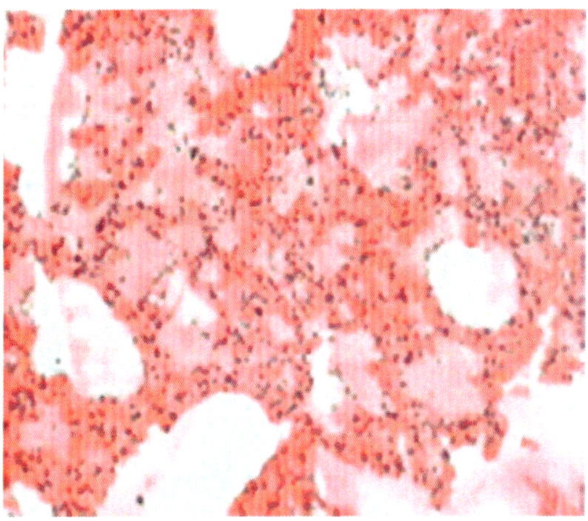

Fig. 4.13: Photomicrograph of lung showing oedematous fluid in alveoli

Etiology

- Bacteria.
- Virus.
- Allergy.

Macroscopic features

- Lungs become enlarged.
- Weight of lungs increases.
- Cut surface releases fluid and frothy exudate in trachea and/or bronchi.

Microscopic features

- Serous fluid accumulation in alveoli of lungs
- Fluid may also be seen in some bronchi/ bronchioles.
- Infiltration of inflammatory cells.
- Congestion of lungs.

Pneumonia

Pneumonia is the inflammation of lungs characterized by congestion and consolidation of lungs. Clinically, it is manifested by dyspnoea, coughing, weakness and nasal discharge (Fig. 4.14 A & B). The pathological lesions in lungs are produced in a similar way irrespective of the type of etiological agent and includes various stages like congestion, red hepatization, grey hepatization and resolution.

Stage of congestion: This stage of lung is characterized by active hyperemia and pulmonary oedema. The capillaries are distended with engorged blood and alveoli are filled with watery serous exudate. This requires 2 minutes to few hours to initiate the congestion.

Stage of red hepatization: This stage of lung is characterized by the consolidation of lungs due to accumulation of blood in blood vessels (congestion). The consolidated lungs are firm and look like liver and hence the name "red hepatization". Such affected lung always sinks in water. Alveoli are filled with serous or serofibrinous exudate giving hardness to lungs. In inflammatory condition, the neutrophils, macrophages and lymphocytes along with erythrocytes infiltrate the affected area of lungs. This stage of red hepatization takes 2 days for development of firmness of lung.

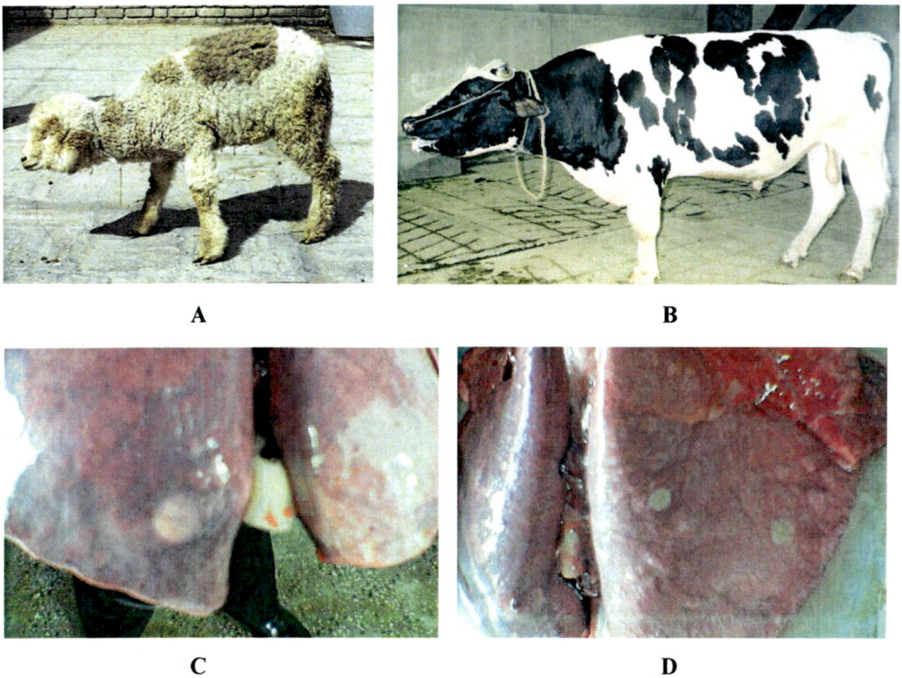

Fig. 4.14: Photograph of lamb (A) showing signs of pneumonia, Severe dyspnoea in Haemorrhagic Septaecemia in Bull(B), Gun shot round lesions in lungs (Sheep pox) (C &D)

Stage of grey hepatization: The lung remains hard but due to lysis and removal of erythrocytes, it becomes grey or less red in colour. Firmness/ hardness of lung remains same and thus, the name grey hepatization. There is increase in infiltration of inflammatory cells like macrophages, lymphocytes, epithelioid cells depending on the virulence of etiological agents.

Stage of resolution: After a week, the recovery starts in the form of resorption of fluid; autolysed cells and debris is removed by phagocytic cells. The causative organism is neutralized or removed from the lungs through immunity of body. After a few days the lung parenchyma becomes normal and starts functioning. If the causative agent is more virulent, it may cause death of animal due to respiratory failure or may cause permanent lesions like formation of scar, carnification, granuloma etc. There are various types of pneumonia caused by bacteria, virus, fungi, parasites, allergens, chemicals and all such affections of lungs are classified as under.

Bronchopneumonia

Bronchopneumonia is the inflammation of lungs involving bronchi or bronchioles along with alveoli. It is thought to be spread through bronchogenous route and is the common type of pneumonia in animals (Figs. 4.15 & 4.16).

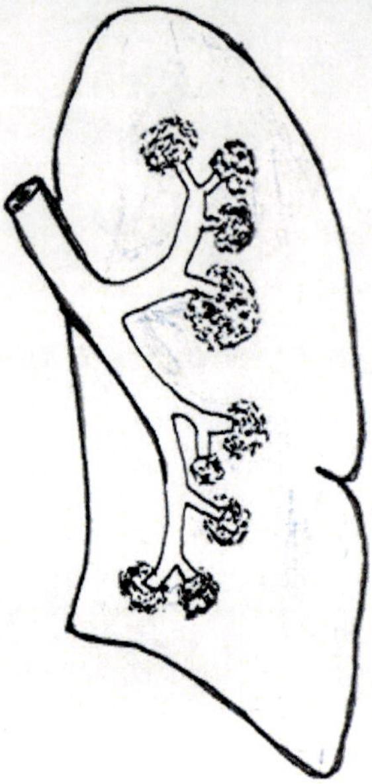

Fig. 4.15: Diagram showing bronchogenous spread of causal agent in lung

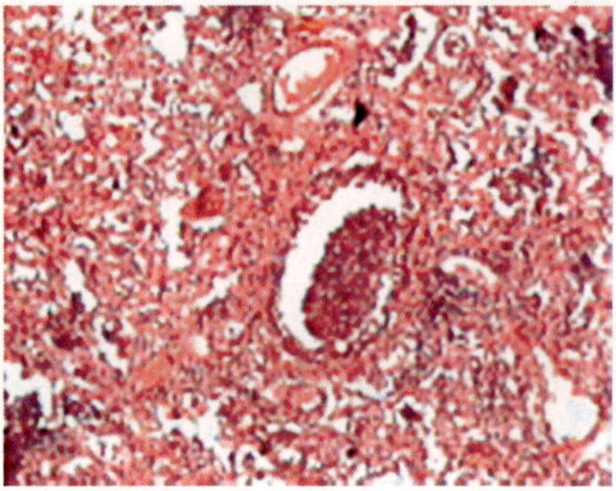

Fig. 4.16: Photomicrograph showing bronchopneumonia

Etiology

- Virus.
- Bacteria.
- Chemicals.
- Mycoplasma.
- Chlamydia.
- Parasites.
- Fungus.
- Mainly through bronchogenous route.

Macroscopic features

- Congestion and consolidation of anterior and ventral parts of lungs (lobular pneumonia).
- Patchy lesions on one or several lobes and adjacent area showing emphysema.
- Mediastinal lymphnodes are swollen.
- Presence of round gun shot like lesions in sheep pox (Fig.4.14 C&D)

Microscopic features

- Congestion, oedema or hemorrhage in lung.
- Infiltration of neutrophils, mononuclear cells in and around bronchioles/ bronchi.
- Catarrhal inflammation of bronchi.
- Proliferation of bronchiolar epithelium.

Interstitial Pneumonia

Interstitial pneumonia is the inflammation of the lungs characterized by thickening of alveolar septa due to serous/fibrinous exudate along with infiltration of neutrophils and/or mononuclear cells and proliferation of fibroblasts. It is also known as lobar pneumonia (Figs. 4.17 & 4.18).

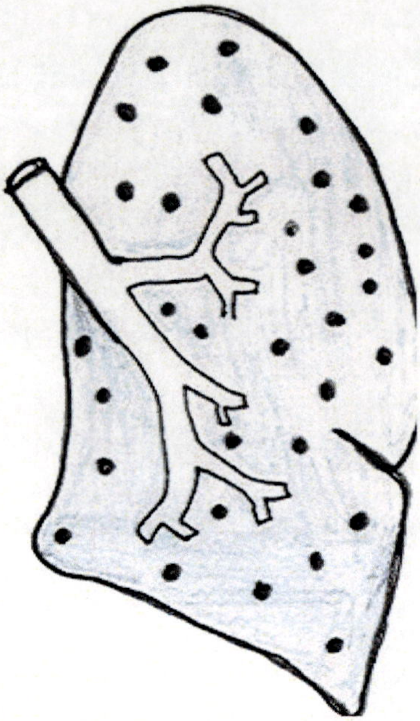

Fig. 4.17: Diagram showing hematogenous spread of causal agent in lung

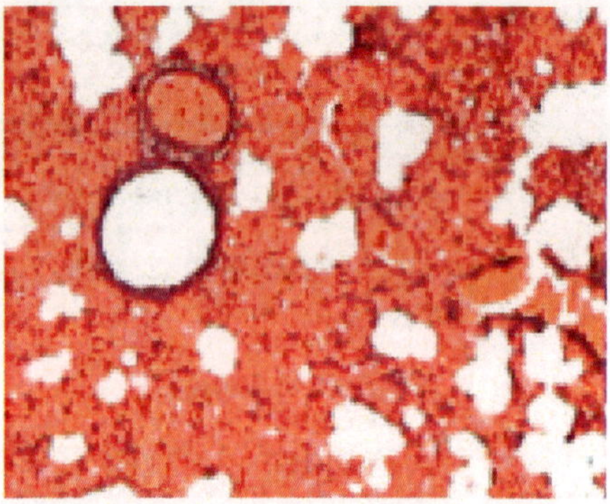

Fig. 4.18: Photomicrograph showing interstitial pneumonia

Etiology

- Bacteria.
- Virus.
- Chlamydia.
- Parasites.
- Mainly through hematogenous route.

Macroscopic features

- Lungs are pale or dark red in colour.
- Oedema, dripping of fluid from cut surface.

Microscopic features

- Alveoli may have serous or fibrinous exudate.
- Thickening of alveolar septa due to accumulation of exudate, inflammatory cells and in chronic cases, proliferation of fibrous tissue.
- Infiltration of mononuclear cells in alveolar septa.

Fibrinous Pneumonia

Fibrinous pneumonia is the inflammation of lungs characterized by the presence of fibrin in alveoli or bronchioles and may give rise to hyaline membrane formation over the surface of alveoli or bronchiole.

Etiology

- Bacteria.
- Virus.
- Parasites.
- Toxin/poisons.

Macroscopic features

- Antero-ventral portion of lung is congested and consolidation.
- Colour of lungs become deep red due to congestion.
- Surface of lungs is covered by fibrin sheet.
- Interlobular septa are prominent due to accumulation of plasma and fibrin.

Microscopic features

- Principal exudate is fibrin, fills alveoli, bronchioles and bronchi (Fig. 4.19).

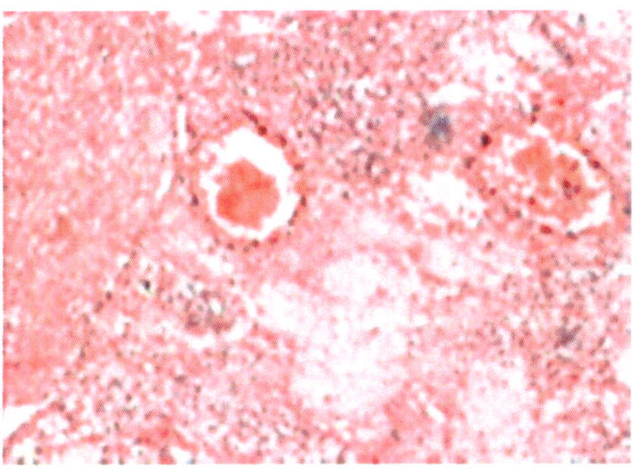

Fig. 4.19: Photomicrograph of fibrinous pneumonia

- Congestion and/or hemorrhage.
- Infiltration of neutrophils, macrophages and giant cells.
- Formation of eosinophilic false membrane of fibrin over the surface of alveoli and bronchiole known as "hyaline membrane pneumonia" (Fig. 4.20).

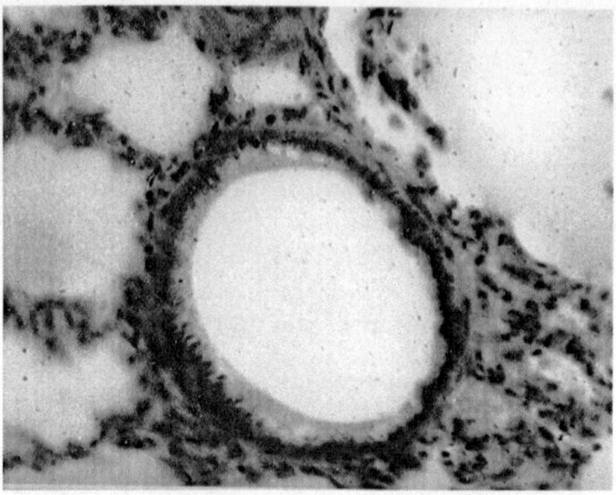

Fig. 4.20: Photomicrograph showing hyaline membrane pneumonia

Verminous Pneumonia

Verminous pneumonia is caused by parasites and is characterized by the presence of lesions of bronchopneumonia along with parasites or their larva (Fig. 4.21).

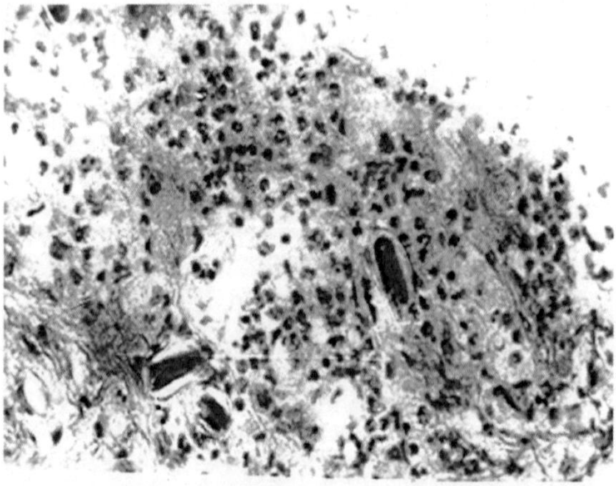

Fig. 4.21: Photomicrograph showing verminous Pneumonia

Etiology

- *Metastrongylus apri* in pig.
- *Dictyocaulus filariae* in sheep and goat.
- *D. viviparus* in cattle and buffaloes.
- *D. arnfieldi* in horse and donkeys.
- *Capillaria aerophila* in dogs and cats.

Macroscopic features

- Multiple petechial hemorrhage in lungs at the site of parasite penetration.
- Mature worms in alveoli, bronchioles and bronchi.
- Mucopurulent exudate in alveoli/bronchi.
- Pulmonary oedema, emphysema.

Microscopic features

- Dilation of bronchiole/ bronchi
- Lesions of chronic suppurative bronchiolitis
- Focal areas of inflammation in the vicinity of parasites and around bronchioles.
- Hyperplasia of bronchiolar epithelium.
- Infiltration of eosinophils and lymphocytes.

Aspiration Pneumonia

Aspiration pneumonia is caused by faulty medication through drenching which reaches lungs instead of targetted place (digestive tract) and characterized by necrosis and gangrene of lung parenchyma.

Etiology

- Drugs, food, foreign body and oil drench which reaches in lungs through trachea.
- Paresis of throat predisposes the animal for aspiration pneumonia.

Macroscopic features

- Congestion and consolidation of anterior and ventral portion of lung.
- Affected part becomes green/ black in colour, moist gangrene.

- Affected lungs are often foul smelling.
- Presence of foreign body like heads of wheats, parts of corn, oil, milk etc.

Microscopic features

- Thrombosis of blood vessels.
- Necrosis in lungs.
- Presence of saprophytes, leucocytes and bacteria cause liquefaction and gangrene.
- Gangrenous lesions surrounded by intense inflammation (Fig. 4.22).

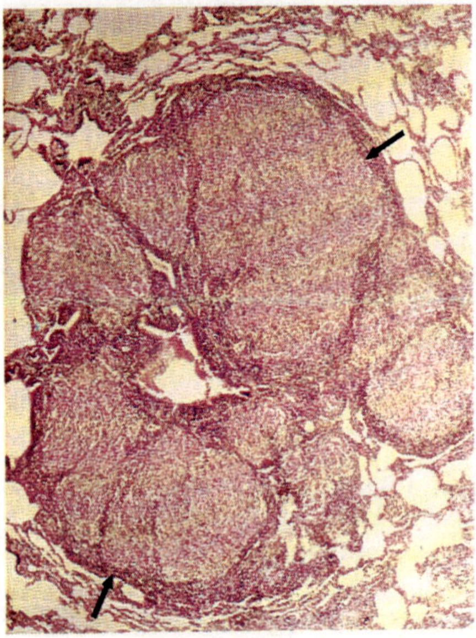

Fig. 4.22: Photomicrograph showing aspiration pneumonia

- Congestion.

Mycotic Pneumonia

Mycotic pneumonia is caused by a variety of fungi and characterized by the presence of chronic granulomatous lesions in lungs (Figs. 4.23 & 4.24).

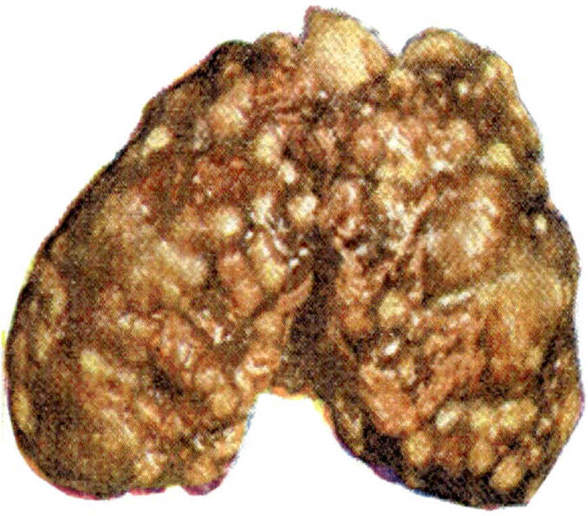

Fig. 4.24: Photomicrograph showing mycotic pneumonia

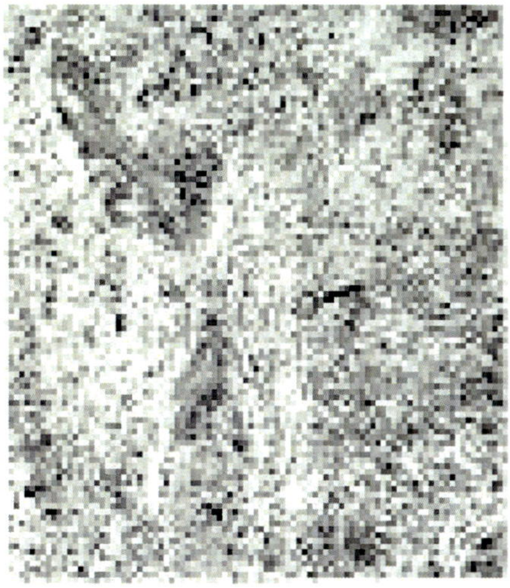

Fig. 4.24: Photograph showing mycotic pneumonia

Etiology

- *Aspergillus fumigatus*.
- *Blastomyces* sp.
- *Cryptococcus* sp.
- *Coccidioidomyces immitis*.

Macroscopic features

- Nodules in lungs.
- On cut, cheese-like caseative mass comes out from nodules.
- Caseation involves both bronchiole and alveoli.
- Such lesions may also be present in trachea, bronchi and air sacs.

Microscopic features

- Presence of granulomatus lesions i.e. caseative necrosis, macrophages, epithelioid cells, lymphocytes, giant cells, fibroblasts etc.
- Presence of branched hyphae of fungi in the necrosed area.

Tuberculous Pneumonia

Tuberculous pneumonia is caused by Mycobacterium sp. and is characterized by the presence of chronic granulomatous lesions in the lungs (Figs. 4.25 to 4.29).

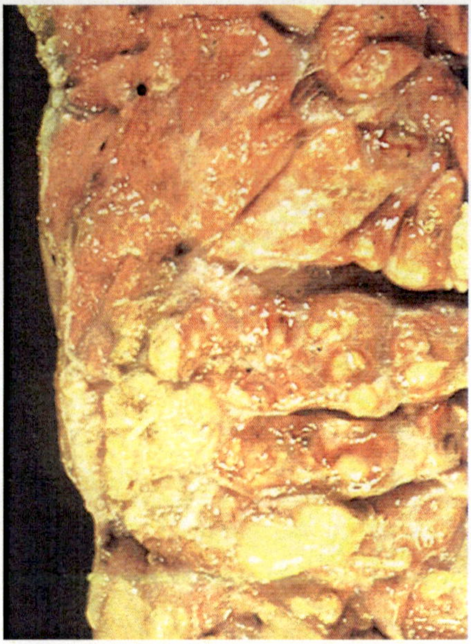

Fig. 4.25: Photograph of lung showing tubercle/granulomatous lesion

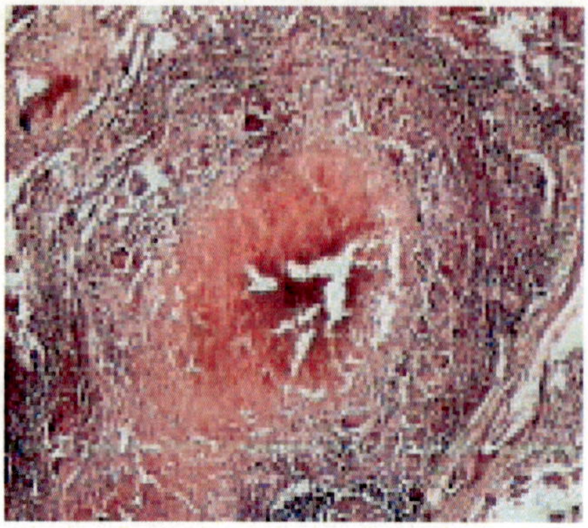

Fig. 4.26: Photomicrograph of lung showing. tubercle

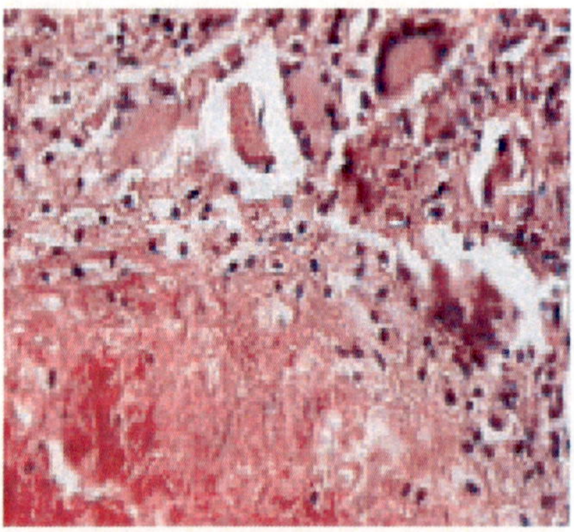

Fig. 4.27: Photomicrograph of lung showing granulomatous lesions

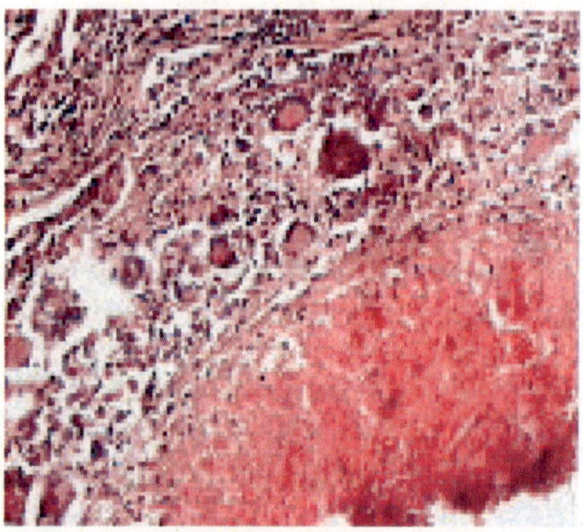

Fig. 4.28: Photomicrograph of lung showing granulomatous lesions and giant cells

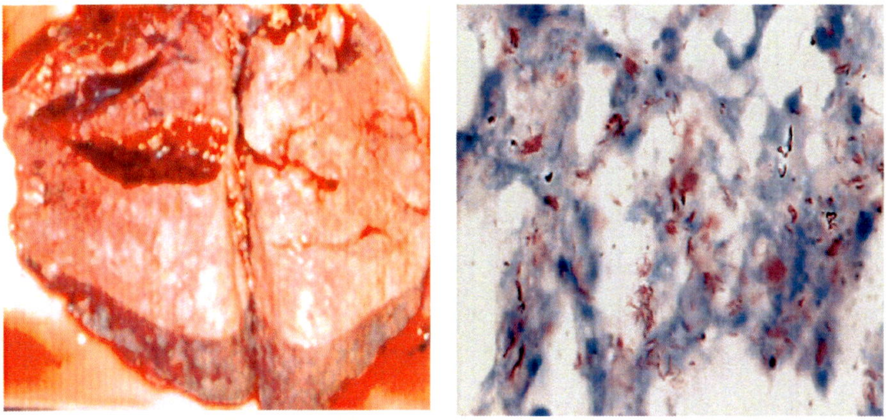

(1) (2)

Fig.4.29: Tuberculous pneumonia (1) Tuberculous nodules in lungs, and (2) acid-fast bacilli in lung tissue section

Etiology

- Mycobacterium tuberculosis.
- M. bovis.

Macroscopic features

- Grey, white or light yellowish nodules in lungs.
- Nodules are hard, painful and/or calcified.
- Animal carcass is cachectic, weak or emaciated.
- On cut, the cheesy material comes out from the nodules.

Microscopic features

- Presence of tubercle/granuloma in lungs which comprises a central necrosed area surrounded by macrophages, epithelioid cells, lymphocytes, Langhan's giant cells and covered by fibrous covering.
- Acid-fast rod shaped bacteria may be present in necrosed area.
- Central area may be calcified.

Table 4.1: Differential features of various types of Pneumonia

	Bronchopneum Onia	**Interstitial**	**Fibrinous**	**Verminous**	**Aspiration**	**Mycotic**	**Tuberculous**
Macroscopic features	1. Congestion and Consolidation of anterior and ventral parts of lungs (Lobular pneumonia). 2. Patchy lesions on one or several lobes and adjacent area shows emphysema. 3. Mediastinal lymphnodes are swollen.	1. Lungs are pale or dark red in colour. 2. Oedema, dripping of fluid from cut surface	1. Antero-ventral portion of lung is congested and consolidated. 2. Colour of lungs become deep red due to congestion 3. Surface of lungs is covered by fibrin sheet. 4. Interlobular septa are prominent due to accumulation of plasma and fibrin.	1. Multiple petechial haemorrhage in lungs at the site of parasite penetration. 2. Mature worms in alveoli, bronchioles and bronchi. 3. Mucopurulent exudate in alveoli/ bronchi. 4. Pulmonary oedema, emphysema.	1. Congestion and consolidation of anterior and ventral portion of lung. 2. Affected part becomes green/ black in colour, moist gangrene. 3. Affected lungs are often foul smelling. 4. Presence of foreign body like heads of wheats, parts of corn, oil, milk etc.	1. Nodules in lungs 2. On cut, cheese like caseative mass comes out from nodules. 3. Caseation involves both bronchiole and alveoli. 4. Such lesions may also present in trachea, bronchi and air sacs.	1. Grey, white or light yellowish nodules in lungs. 2. Nodules are hard, painful and/or calcified. 3. Animal carcass is cachectic, weak or emaciated. 4. On cut, the cheesy material comes out from the nodules.

	Bronchopneum Onia	Interstitial	Fibrinous	Verminous	Aspiration	Mycotic	Tuberculous
Microscopic features	1. Congestion, oedema or haemorrhage in lung. 2. Infiltration of neutrophils, mononuclear cells in and around bronchioles/ bronchi. 3. Catarrhal inflammation of bronchi. 4. Proliferation of bronchiolar epithelium	1. Alveoli may have serous or fibrinous exudate. 2. Thickening of alveolar septa due to accumulation of exudate, inflammatory cells and in chronic cases, proliferation of fibrous tissue. 3. Infiltration of mononuclear cells in alveolar septa.	1. Principal exudate is fibrin, fills alveoli, bronchioles and bronchi. 2. Congestion and/or haemorrhages 3. Infiltration of neutrophils, macrophages and giant cells 4. Formation of eosinophilic false membrane of fibrin over the surface of alveoli and bronchiole and then known as “hyaline membrane pneumonia”.	1. Dilation of bronchiole/ bronchi 2. Lesions of chronic suppurative bronchiolitis 3. Focal areas of inflammation in the vicinity of parasites and around bronchioles. 4. Hyperplasia of bronchiolar epithelium. 5. Infiltration of eosinophils and lymphocytes.	1. Thrombosis of blood vessels. 2. Necrosis in lungs. 3. Presence of saprophytes, leucocytes and bacteria cause liquefaction and gangrene. 4. Gangrenous lesions surrounded by intense inflammation 5. Congestion	1. Presence of granulomatus lesions i.e. caseative necrosis, macrophages, epithelioid cells, lymphocytes, giant cells, fibroblasts etc. 2. Presence of branched hyphae of fungi in the necrosed area.	1. Presence of tubercle/ granul oma in lungs which comprises a central necrosed area surrounded by macrophages, epithelioid cells, lymphocytes, Langhan’s giant cells and covered by fibrous covering. 2. Acid-fast rod shaped bacteria may present in necrosed area. 3. Central area may be calcified.

Pulmonary Adenomatosis

Pulmonary adenomatosis is a slow viral disease of sheep and is characterized by metaplasia of alveolar squamous epithelium to cuboidal and /or columnar epithelium leading to glandular appearance of alveoli (Figs. 4.30 & 4.31).

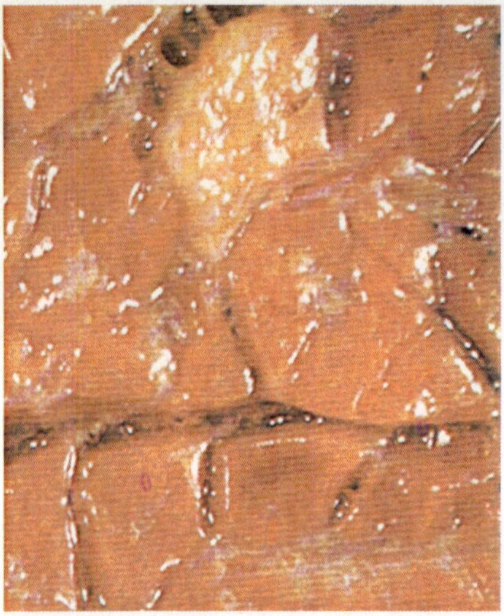

Fig. 4.30: Photograph showing pulmonary adenomatosis

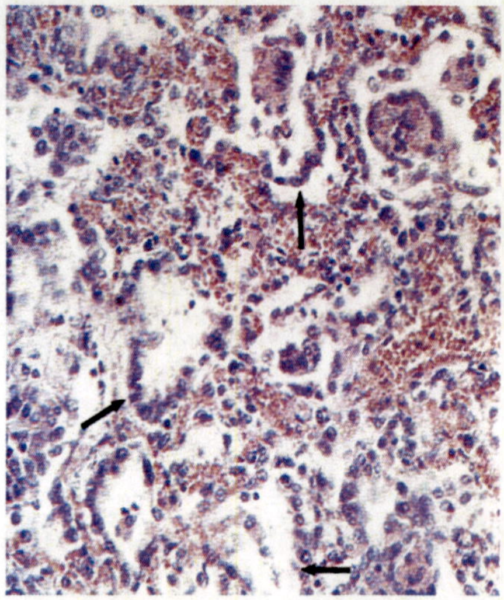

Fig. 4.31: Photomicrograph showing pulmonary adenomatosis

Etiology

- Retrovirus.
- Pulmonary adenomatosis virus.

Macroscopic features

- Multiple focal areas of consolidation in lungs.
- Imprint of ribs on lungs.
- Congestion and hardening of mediastinal lymphnodes.

Microscopic features

- Metaplasia of alveolar epithelium leading to formation of glandular structures in alveoli.
- Metaplasia of simple squamous epithelium to cuboidal or columnar epithelium which gives alveoli a gland like look.

- Mild inflammatory reaction.
- Proliferation of fibrous tissue.

Hypersensitivity Pneumonitis

Hypersensitivity pneumonitis is the inflammation of lung caused by an allergic reaction of antigen (allergen) and characterized by interstitial pneumonia, emphysema, hyaline membrane formation and hyperplasia of alveolar epithelium.

Etiology

- Allergens.
- Parasites – *Dictyocaulus viviparous*.
- Moldy hay.
- Fungus – *Aspergillus* sp.

Macroscopic features

- Lobes may contain small grey foci.
- Presence of yellow and dense mucus in lumen of bronchi.
- Excessive accumulation of air in lungs due to emphysema.
- Presence of worms/larvae.

Microscopic features

- Extensive infiltration of lymphocytes, monocytes and eosinophils around the bronchi and bronchioles.
- Accumulation of catarrhal exudate in bronchi/ bronchiole.
- Emphysema as a result of widening of alveoli.
- Hyperplasia of bronchiolar musculature.
- Inflammatory cells in interalveolar septa may form small granulomas.
- Formation of hyaline membrane over alveolar and bronchiolar epithelium.

Pneumoconiasis

Pneumoconiasis is the granulomatous inflammation of lungs caused by aerogenous dust particles of sand, silica, beryllium, carbon or asbestos. It is also known as anthracosis (Figs. 4.32 & 4.33).

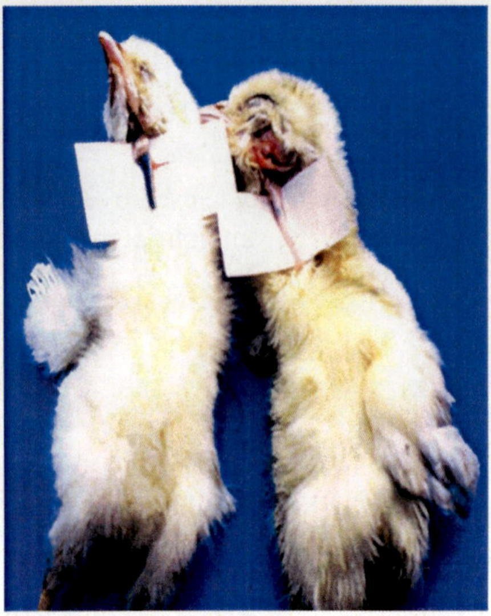

Fig. 4.32: Photograph showing deposition of carbon particles in trachea in chicks

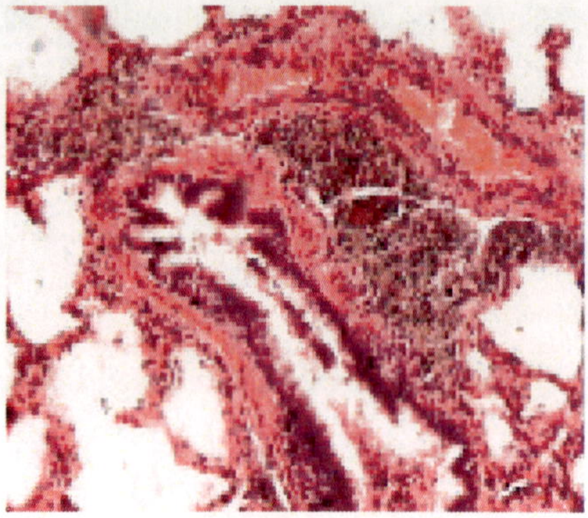

Fig. 4.33: Photomicrograph showing pneumoconiasis

Etiology

- Silica.
- Asbestos.
- Beryllium.
- Bauxite.
- Graphite.
- Carbon.
- Bronchogenous/aerogenous administration of particles inhaled with air, mostly around mines/factories.
- Generator smoke.

Macroscopic features

- Dense fibrous nodules in lungs.
- Presence of carbon particles in trachea/bronchi mixed with mucous exudate.

Microscopic features

- Granuloma formation around the particles of silica/asbestos infiltrated by macrophages, lymphocytes and giant cells
- Silica produces cellular reaction 'Silicosis'.
- Beryllium granuloma looks like tubercule without caseation.
- Asbestosis is characterized by the presence of club shaped filaments bearing cells in lesion.

Pathology of Air Sacs

Air Sacculitis

Air sacculitis is inflammation of air sacs caused by *E. coli*, Mycoplasma, reovirus etc. and characterized by thickening of the wall of air sacs and presence of cheesy exudate (Fig. 4.34).

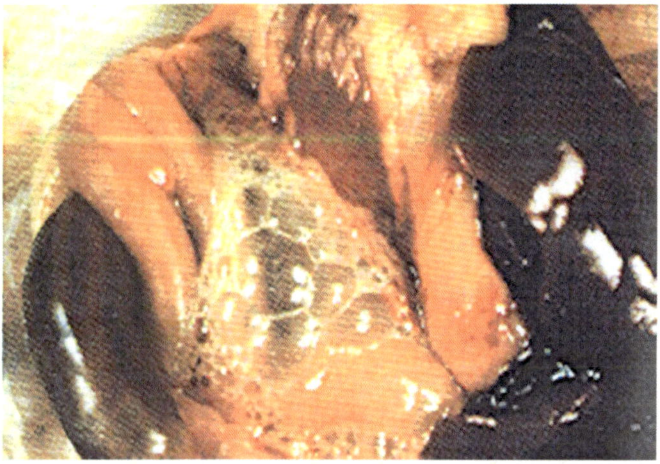

Fig. 4.34: Photograph showing air sacculitis in poultry

Etiology

- Escherichia coli.
- *Mycoplasma gallisepticum.*
- Avian reovirus.

Macroscopic features

- Thickening of the air sac wall, which becomes dirty and cloudy.
- Presence of cheesy exudate in air sacs, congestion of lungs.
- Fibrinous pericarditis.
- Liver is covered with thin fibrinous membrane.

Microscopic features

- Oedema and infiltration of neutrophils and lymphocytes in air sacs.
- Caseous exudate in lungs and air sacs.

Pathology of Pleura

Pleuritis

Pleuritis is the inflammation of pleura characterized by serous, fibrinous or purulent exudate. It is also known as pleurisy.

Etiology

- Mycobacterium tuberculosis.
- Mycoplasma mycoides.
- Haemophilus suis.
- Organisms responsible for pneumonia/ traumatic pericarditis may also cause pleuritis.

Macroscopic features

- Congestion of pleura.
- Serous, fibrinous or purulent exudate.
- Accumulation of clear fluid in pleura/thoracic cavity is called as hydrothorax.
- Presence of blood in thoracic cavity is known as Hemothorax.
- Suppurative exudate in thoracic cavity is known as pyothorax.
- Presence of air in pleural cavity is termed as pneumothorax, while presence of lymph in pleural cavity is called as chylothorax.
- Tuberculous pleuritis is characterized by small nodules on pleura and is known as "***pearly disease***".

- In chronic cases, development of fibrous tissue causes adhesions and is known as adhesive pleuritis.

Microscopic features

- Congestion of blood vessels.
- Infiltration of neutrophils and lymphocytes.
- Thickening of pleura due to oedema.
- Proliferation of fibroblasts producing adhesive lesions.

5

Pathology of Digestive System

Developmental Anomalies

Epitheliogenesis imperfecta of tongue

Abnormal smooth surface of tongue due to small filiform papillae. It occurs as a defect in autosomal recessive gene and occurs in Holstein-Friesian cattle. This is also known as smooth tongue.

Cleft palate

This is most common congenital abnormality that occurs due to failure of oral-nasal cavity to divide leaving cleft. It may also extend towards lips producing 'harelip' condition.

Mega colon

There is distention of colon which abruptly terminates in rectum due to mutant gene in dogs.

Duplication of colon

In dog, the colon is duplicated from caecum to rectum and this defect is associated with malformation in the body of vertebrae T_4 and T_5.

Atresia coli

In calf, the absence of colon occurs and the intestine terminates in blind caecum.

Atresia ani

This is absence of anal opening.

Pathology of Mouth Cavity

Stomatitis

Stomatitis in the inflammation of mucosa of oral cavity (Figs. 5.1 to 5.6). It includes:

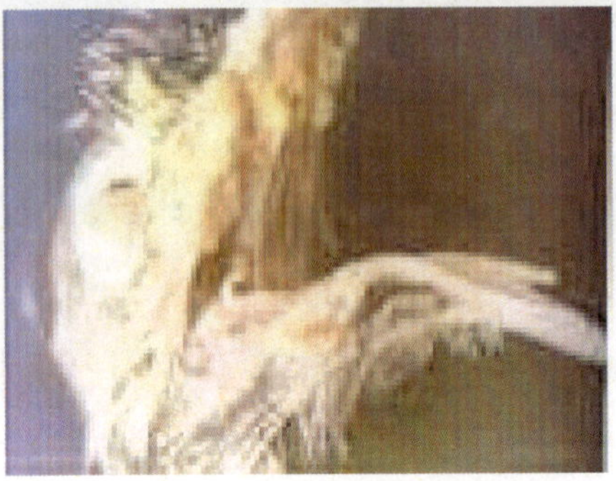

Fig. 5.1: Photograph of mouth cavity of a bird showing stomatitis due to avian pox

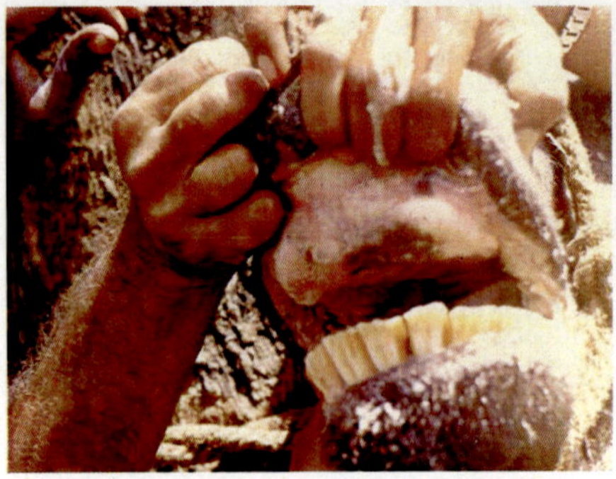

Fig. 5.2: Photograph of mouth cavity of a buffalo having erosive palatitis

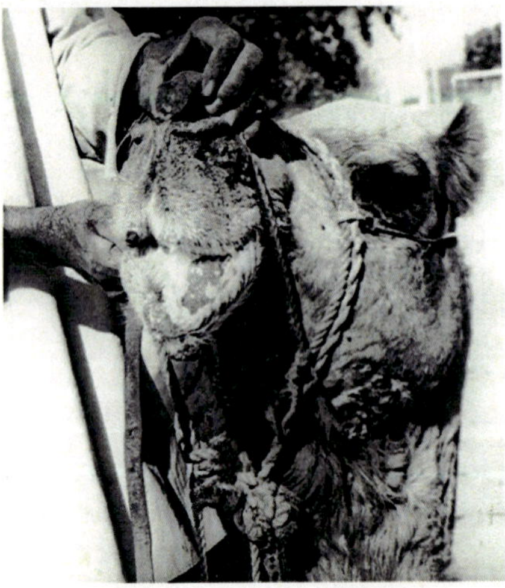

Fig. 5.3: Photograph of mouth of a camel showing cheilitis

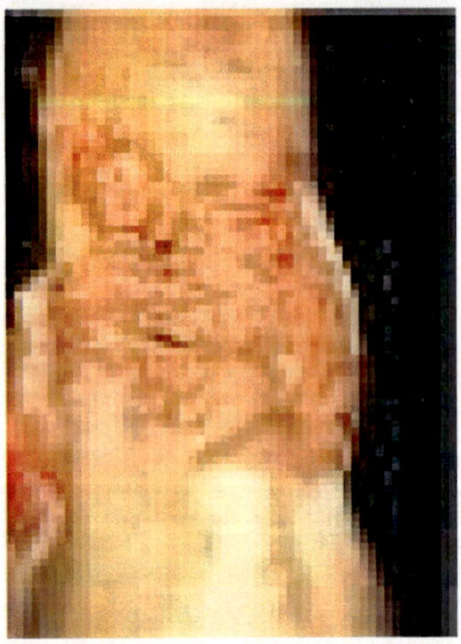

Fig. 5.4: Photograph of tongue showing granulomatous lesions

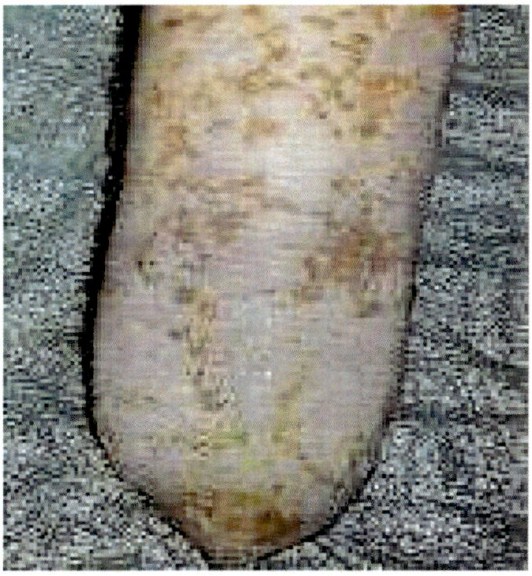

Fig. 5.5: Photograph of tongue showing ulcerative glossitis

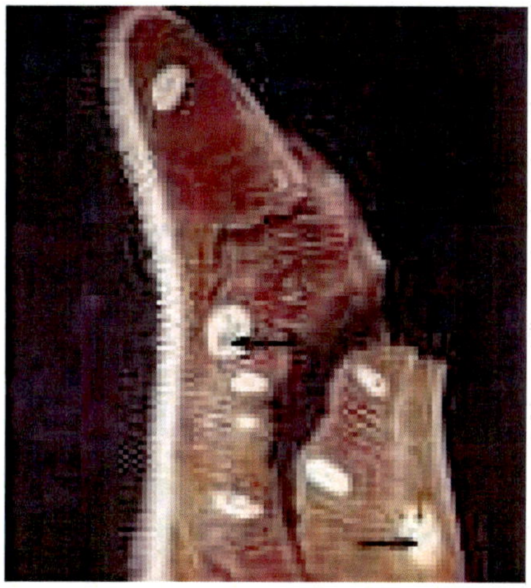

Fig. 5.6: Photograph of tongue showing glossitis due to cysticercosis.

Gingivitis: Inflammation of gums. Glossitis: Inflammation of tongue. Cheilitis: Inflammation of lips.

Tonsilitis: Inflammation of tonsil. Palatitis/Lampas: Inflammation of palates.

Etiology

- Trauma due to nails, wire, or any sharp object like needle.
- Physical due to hot milk, medicines etc.
- Chemical – Alkali / acids.
- Microorganisms – Bacteria, virus, fungi.

Macroscopic features

- Catarrhal stomatitis: Mucous exudation in oral cavity.
- Vesicular stomatitis: Vesicles in oral mucosal e.g. FMD.
- Erosive stomatitis: Erosions in oral mucosa e.g. Rinderpest.
- Fibrinous stomatitis: False membrane in oral mucosa.
- Ulcerative stomatitis: Presence of ulcers in oral mucosa e.g. mucosal disease.

Microscopic features

- Congestion of oral mucosa.
- Presence of erosions, vesicles or ulcers.

- Infiltration of neutrophils, lymphocytes and macrophages.
- Presence of fibrinous exudate in the form of diphtheritic membrane.

Pathology of Oesophagus and Crop Choke

Choke is complete or partial obstruction of oesophagus either due to any foreign material or pressure from adjoining areas (Fig. 5.7).

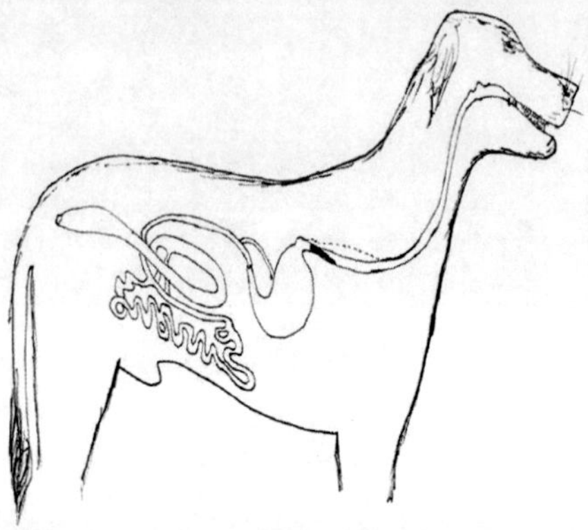

Fig. 5.7: Diagram of alimentary tract of dog showing choke in oesophagus due to bone

Etiology

- Beets, turnip, carrots, bone.
- Abscess, tumor of neck area.

Macroscopic features

- Tympany.
- Gangrene, sapremia and toxaemia.
- Sac-like dilatation "Oesophageal diverticulum"
- Perforation due to sharp bone ends.

Microscopic features

- Necrosis gangrene at a point of obstruction.
- Congestion hemorrhage in perforated cases.

Oesophagitis

Oesophagitis is the inflammation of oesophagus caused by trauma, parasites etc. and is characterized by catarrhal inflammation, ulceration or stenosis due to fibrosis.

Etiology

- Trauma due to foreign bodies.
- Chemicals – Acids, alkalies.
- Infection – Mucosal disease virus.
- Parasite – *Spirocerca lupi*, sarcosporidiosis (Fig. 5.8).
- Nutritional – Vit. A deficiency.

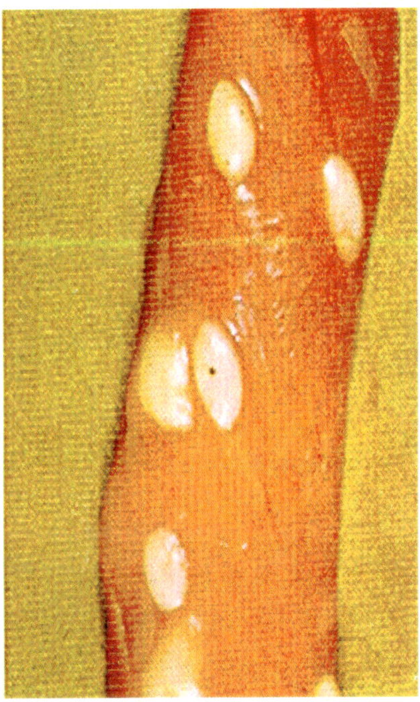

Fig. 5.8: Photograph of oesophagus showing presence of cysts due to sarcosporidiosis

Macroscopic features

- Congestion.
- Ulcer formation (Fig. 5.9).

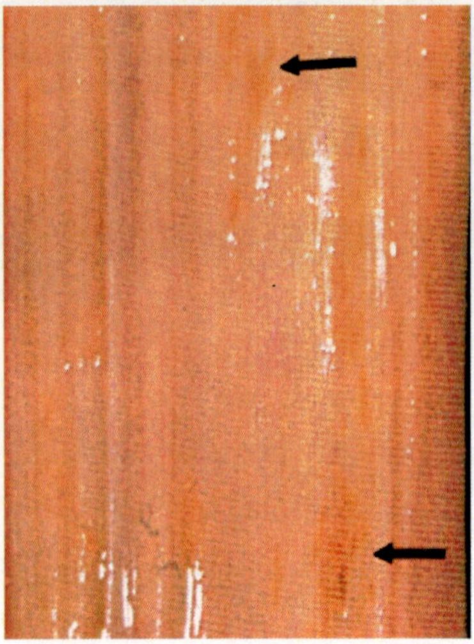

Fig. 5.9: Photograph showing ulcerative esophagitis due to bovine viral diarrhoea virus

- Red streaks of catarrhal inflammation.
- Stenosis due to fibrous nodules or inflammatory exudate.
- Enlargement of glands due to Vit A. defi. (Fig. 5.10).

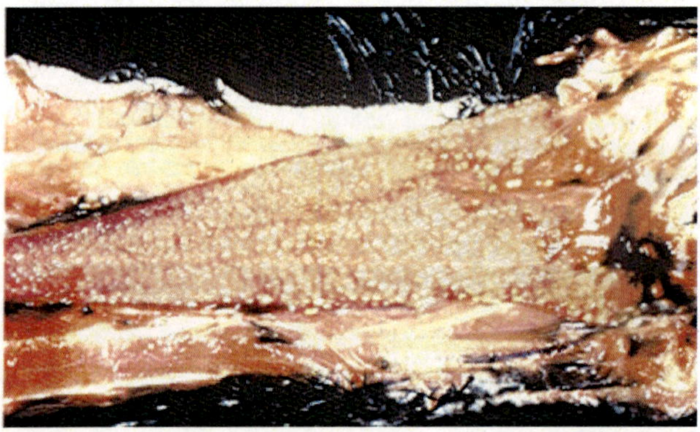

Fig. 5.10: Photograph of oesophagus showing nutritional roup

Microscopic features

- Congestion, hemorrhage.
- Ulceration.

- Infiltration of neutrophils, lymphocytes.
- Sub-epithelial fibrosis/nodules by *Spirocerea lupi*.

Ingluvitis

Ingluvitis is the inflammation of crop caused by fungi and characterized by ulcerative or diphtheritic lesions (Fig. 5.11).

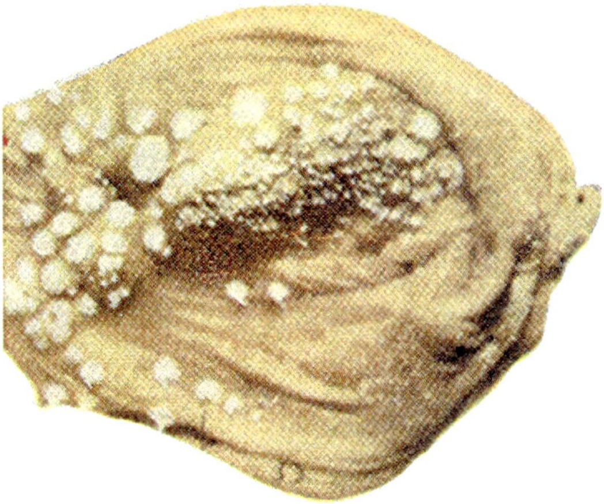

Fig. 5.11: Photograph of crop showing ingluvitis

Etiology

- Candida albicans.
- Monilia albicans.

Macroscopic features

- Turkis towl-like appearance in crop mucosa.
- Round and raised ulcers.
- In moniliasis, formation of diphtheritic membrane.

Microscopic features

- Necrotic and ulcerative lesions.
- Fibrinous inflammation with infiltration of mononuclear cells.

Pathology of Stomach

Tympany

Tympany is accumulation of gases in rumen due to failure of eructation as a result of obstruction or due to excessive production of gases characterized by distended rumen and dyspnoea. It is also known as bloat (Fig. 5.12).

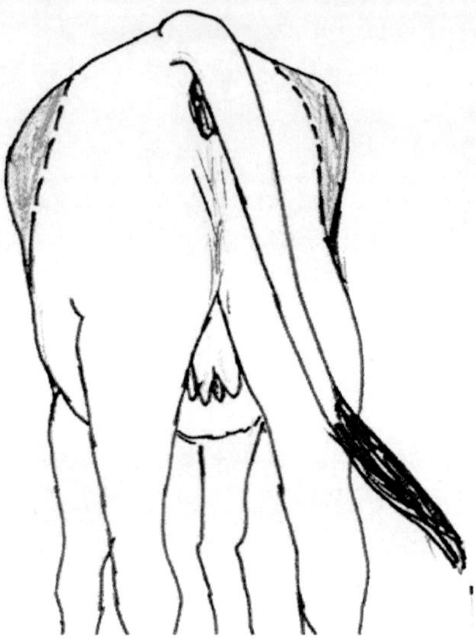

Fig. 5.12: Diagram showing tympany in a cow

Etiology

- Choke of oesophagus.
- Sudden change in animal feed with high content of legumes.
- Excessive lush green fodder.

Macroscopic features

- Rumen is distended due to excessive accumulation of gases (CO_2, H_2S, CO).
- Distended rumen compresses diaphragm to hinder respiration.
- Tarry colour blood, pale liver and rupture of diaphragm.
- On rupture of rumen gas comes out (dry tympany).
- The gas is trapped in small bubbles in the ruminal fluid forming foams

and is not easily removed. This is known as “frothy bloat”, which is produced by saponin and water soluble proteins and due to reduction in surface tension in the absence of fatty acids that favours froth formation.

Microscopic features

- Haemorrhage in lungs, pericardium, trachea and lymphnodes.
- Atelectasis in lungs.

Rumenitis

Rumenitis is the inflammation of rumen in ruminant animals caused by change in diet, chemicals or drugs and characterized by seropurulent exudate or ulcer formation with or without parakeratosis.

Etiology

- Change in diet, corn or alfaalfa hay.
- Chemicals/drugs e.g. potassium antimony tartrate.
- *Spherophorus necrophorus* infection

Macroscopic features

- Ulcers.
- Spherical white nodules of 1-2 cm diameter size.
- Sloughing of mucosa.

Microscopic features

- Seropurulent exudate.
- Ulcers.
- Infiltration of lymphocytes and neutrophils.
- Fibrous nodules due to hyperplasia of fibroblasts.
- Parakeratosis.

Reticulitis

Reticulitis is the inflammation of reticulum in ruminant animals caused by trauma/perforation by foreign body including sharp object like needles, wires, etc. and characterized by abscess formation, adhesions, peritonitis and pericarditis (Fig. 5.13).

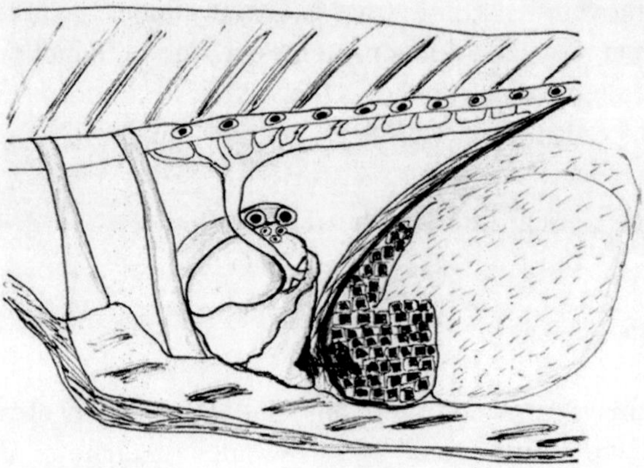

Fig. 5.13: Diagram showing penetration of needle from reticulum (Traumatic reticulitis)

Etiology

- Foreign body – sharp objects like needles, wires etc.

Macroscopic features

- Perforation of reticulum by foreign body.
- Abscessation/suppuration.
- Peritonitis, adhesions of reticulum with diaphragm.
- Pericarditis due to foreign body (traumatic reticulo pericarditis).

Microscopic features

- Infiltration of neutrophils, macrophages, lymphocytes.
- Proliferation of fibroblasts producing adhesions.
- Liquefactive necrosis.

Omasitis

Omasitis is the inflammation of omasum in ruminant animals caused by *Actinobacillus* sp. and characterized by granulomatous inflammatory reaction.

Etiology

- *Actinobacillus ligneiresi.*

Macroscopic features

- Granulomatous nodules in omasum.

Microscopic features

- Typical granuloma formation.
- Sulphur granules of Actinobacillus in the centre of lesion.

Abomasitis

Abomasitis is the inflammation of abomasum in ruminants caused by chemicals/drugs, bacteria, virus or parasites and characterized by congestion, oedema and/or hemorrhagic ulcers (Fig. 5.14 to 5.16).

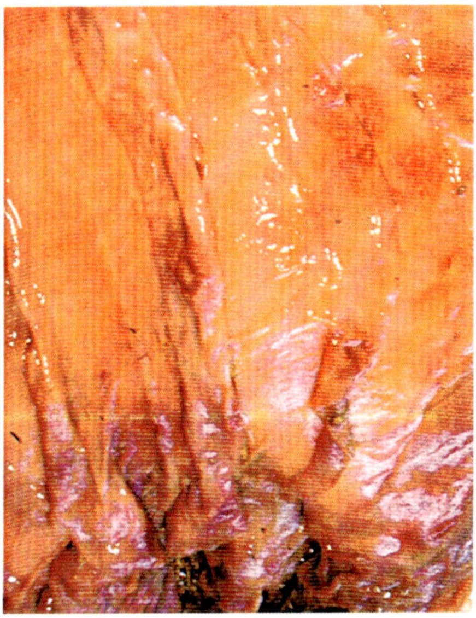

Fig. 5.14: Photograph showing ulcerative abomasitis

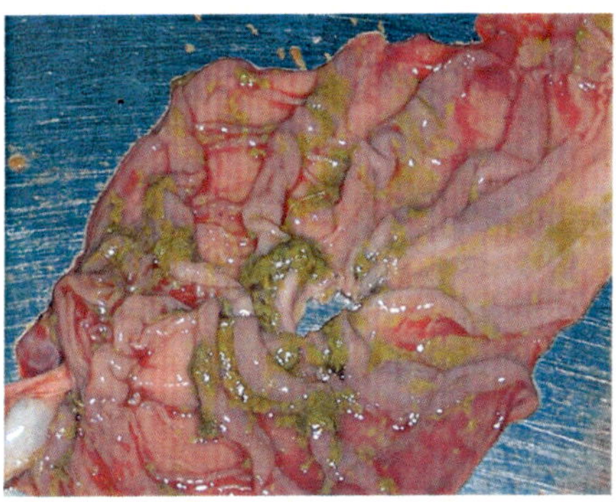

Fig. 5.15: Abomasum showing oedema and congestion leading to thickening of abomasal folds

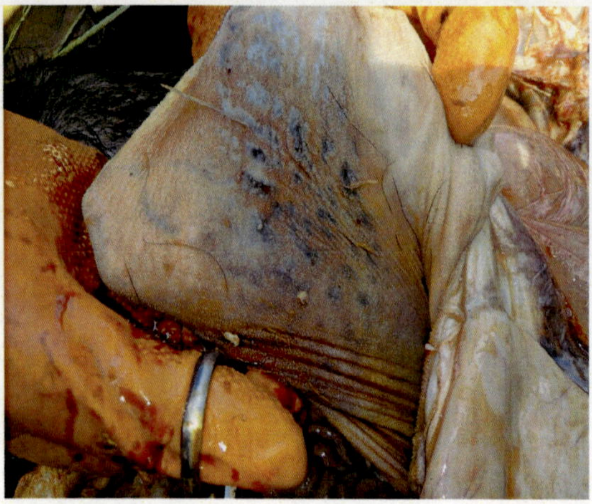

Fig. 5.16: Photograph showing punched out ulcers in abomasum

Etiology

- Chemicals/drugs.
- Bacteria e.g. *Clostridium septicum* cause of braxy.
- Virus e.g. Hog cholera, mucosal disease.
- Parasites e.g. *Theileria* sp.

Macroscopic features

- Presence of ulcers (button ulcers in Hog cholera).
- Congestion, oedema of abomasal folds, hemorrhage in braxy.

Microscopic features

- Catarrhal, hemorrhagic abomasits.
- Presence of Gram positive rods in case of braxy.
- Neutrophilic and lymphocytic infiltration.
- Congestion and hemorrhage.
- Ulceration with lymphocytic infiltration.

Impaction of Rumen and Reticulum

Impaction of rumen and reticulum is common in cattle and buffaloes. It is caused by heavy carbohydrate diet and characterized by atony of rumen, indigestion, acidosis and hemorrhage on serous membranes.

Etiology

- Overfeeding of carbohydrate feed.
- Lack of water.
- Defective teeth or damaged tongue.
- Paralysis of rumen.

Macroscopic features

- Atony of rumen due to lactic acid production.
- Rumen is filled with hard, caked undigested food with foul odour.
- Hemoconcentration, anuria, blood becomes dark in colour.

Microscopic features

- Haemorrhage in lungs.
- Desquamation of ruminal epithelium.
- Lesions of acidosis/toxicosis.

Gastritis

Gastritis is the inflammation of stomach in non-ruminant animals having simple stomach caused by chemicals/drugs, bacteria, virus, parasite and characterized by congestion, oedema, hemorrhage and ulceration. Inflammation of proventriculus in poultry is termed as proventriculitis (Fig. 5.17).

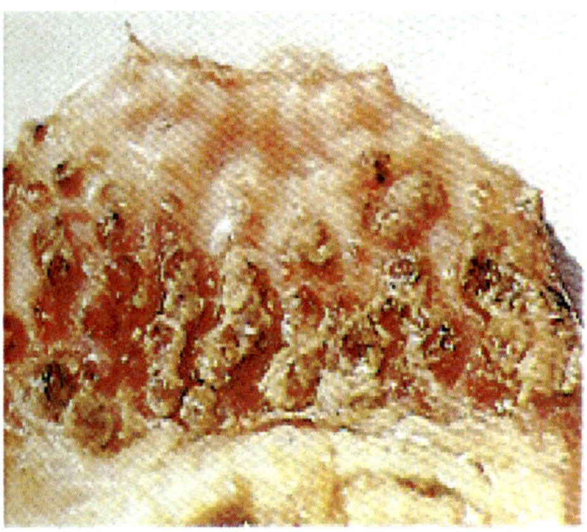

Fig. 5.17: Photograph showing proventriculitis

Etiology

- Physical – overfeeding, trauma.
- Chemicals – Acid/alkali.
- Microorganisms such as bacteria, virus, fungi.
- Parasites e.g. *Trichostrongyles* sp., *Hemonchus* sp.
- Uremia.

Macroscopic features

- Congestion, oedema and haemorrhage of mucosal surface.
- Thick mucous exudate in stomach.
- Presence of vesicles/ulcers on gastric mucosa.

Microscopic features

- Congestion and haemorrhage of gastric mucosa.
- Presence of ulcers/necrosis.
- Infiltration of mononuclear cells.
- Lymphoid hyperplasia.

Pathology of Intestines

Catarrhal Enteritis

- Catarrhal enteritis is characterized by increased number of goblet cells, congestion and infiltration of neutrophils and mononuclear cells in mucosa of intestine (Figs. 5.18 to 5.27).

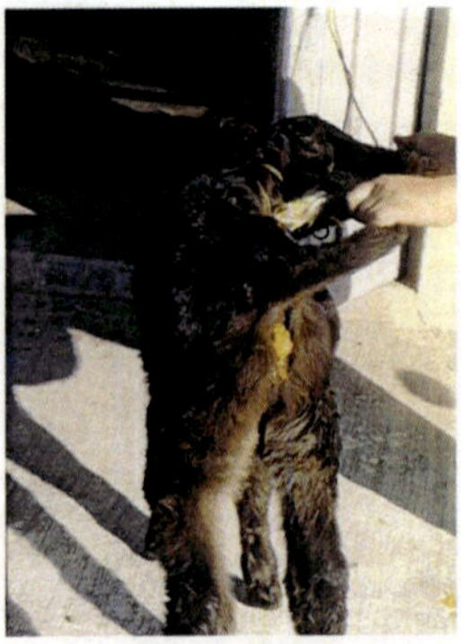

Fig. 5.18: Photograph of calf showing diarrhoea

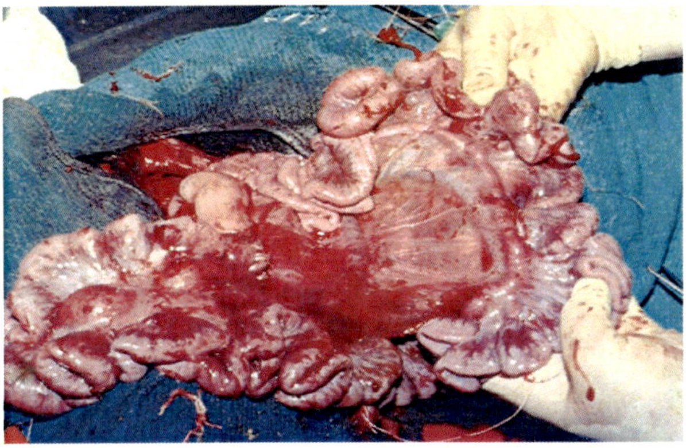

Fig. 5.19: Photograph showing enteritis

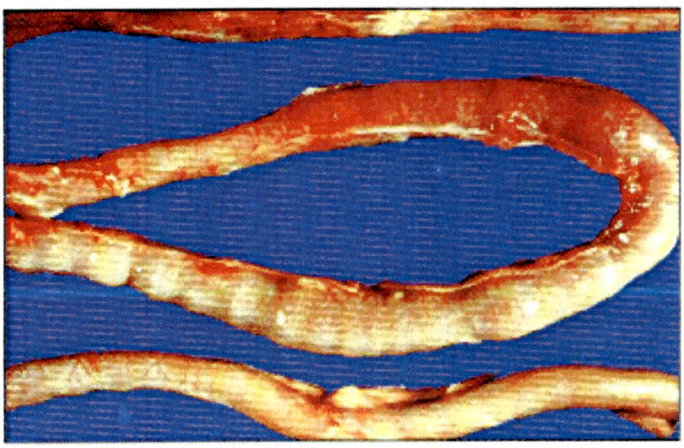

Fig. 5.20: Photograph showing catarrhal enteritis

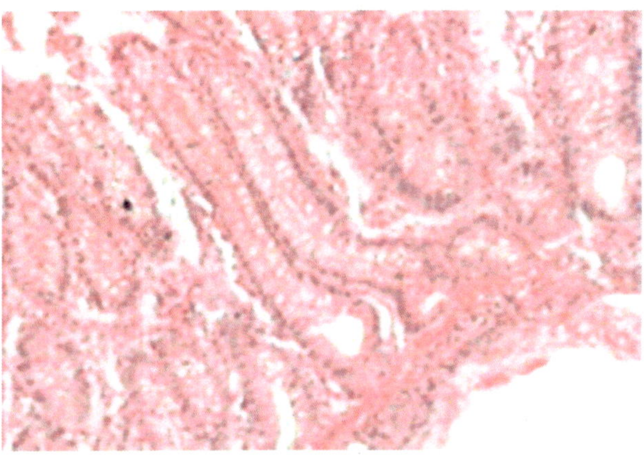

Fig. 5.21: Photomicrograph showing catarrhal enteritis

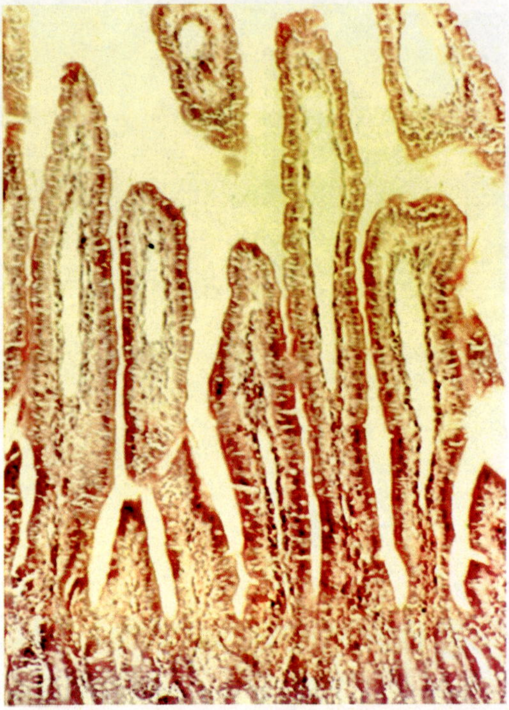

Fig. 5.22: Photomicrograph showing normal length of villi in intestine

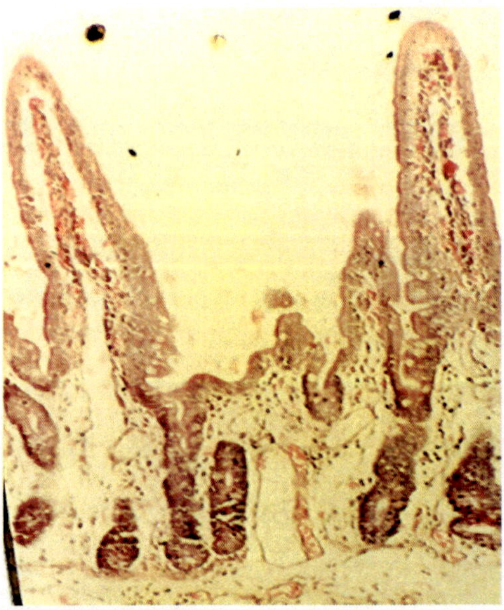

Fig. 5.23: Photomicrograph showing reduced length of villi due to rotavirus infection

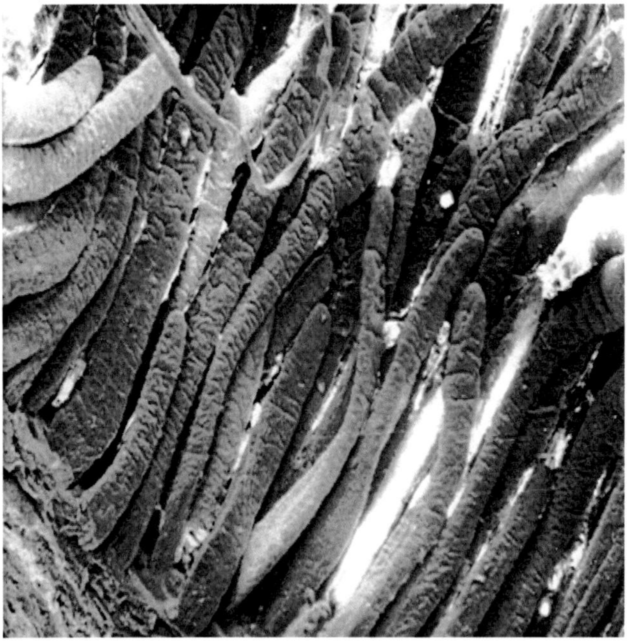

Fig. 5.24: Scanning electron microphotograph showing normal length of villi

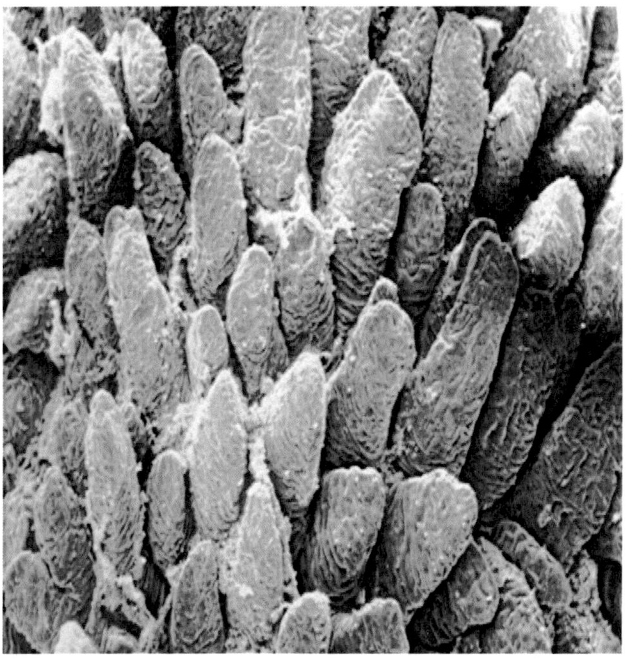

Fig. 5.25: Scanning electron microphotograph showing reduced length of villi with rough surface

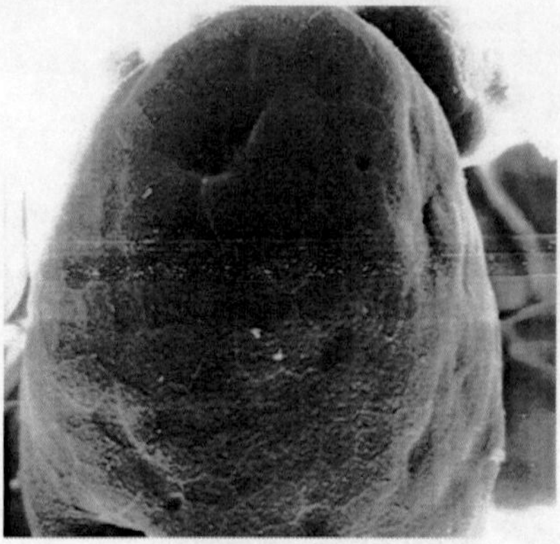

Fig. 5.26: Scanning electron microphotograph showing smooth surface of villi

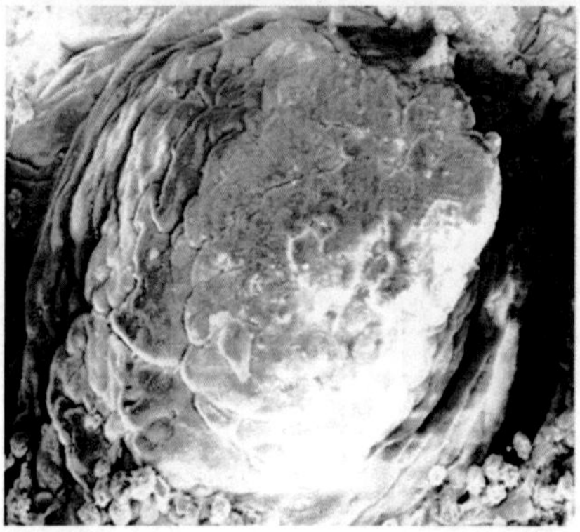

Fig. 5.27: Scanning electron microphotograph showing rough surface of villi

Etiology

- Physical – Foreign bodies and corase feed
- Chemical – drugs
- Microorganisms – *E.coli*, *Salmonella* sp., viruses
- Parasites – *Coccidia*

Macroscopic features

- Presence of catarrhal exudate in lumen of intestine and congestion.
- Thickening of the wall of intestine.
- Diarrhoea.
- Presence of parasites in lumen of intestine.

Microscopic features

- Increased number of goblet cells in intestinal villi, reduced length of villi.
- Congestion.
- Infiltration of polymorphonuclear and mononuclear cells.

Hemorrhagic Enteritis

Hemorrhagic enteritis is characterized by inflammation of the intestines along with hemorrhagic exudate (Figs. 5.28 to 5.30).

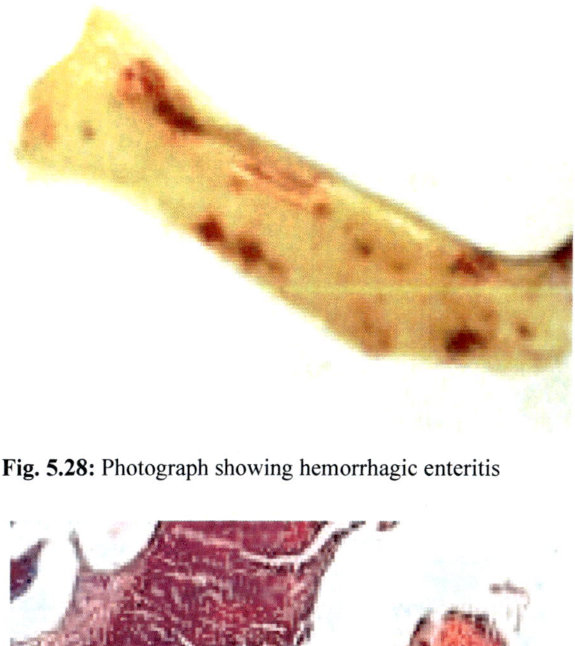

Fig. 5.28: Photograph showing hemorrhagic enteritis

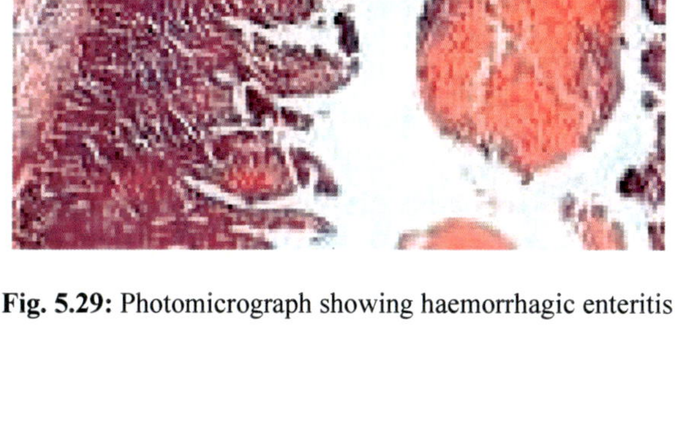

Fig. 5.29: Photomicrograph showing haemorrhagic enteritis

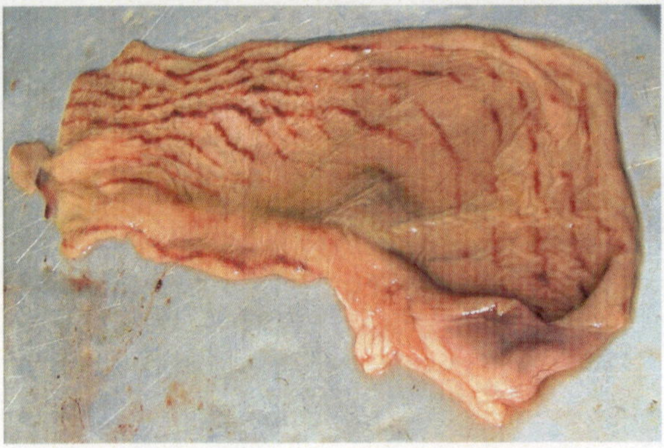

Fig. 5.30: Photograph showing linear haemorrhage (Zebra marking) in large intestine

Etiology

- Bacteria – *E. coli, Bacillus anthracis, Salmonella* sp.
- Virus – Coronavirus, BVD, MD, RP.
- Parasites – *Coccidia*.

Macroscopic features

- Haemorrhagic exudate in intestines; blood mixed intestinal contents.
- Petechial or echymotic hemorrhage in mucosa and submucosa of intestine.
- Presence of erosions/ulcers in mucosa.

Microscopic features

- Hemorrhage in the mucosa of intestine.
- Infiltration of neutrophils and mononuclear cells.
- Erosion or ulcers in intestinal mucosa.
- Presence of coccidia in the mucosa.

Chronic Enteritis

Chronic enteritis is the chronic inflammation of intestine characterized by proliferative changes like proliferation of fibrous tissue, infiltration of mononuclear cells and plasma cells in lamina propria leading to hardening of intestinal wall.

Etiology

- Mycobacterium paratuberculosis in bovines
- Intestinal helminths
- *E. coli* in poultry (Hjarre's disease)

Macroscopic features

- Thickening of the wall of intestine (corrugations in Johne's disease) (Fig. 5.31).
- Thick mucous cover over mucosa of intestine
- Transverse corrugations in the large intestine.
- Granulomatous nodules in duodenum.
- Small, round, raised necrotic foci on serosal surface of intestine covering whole length of intestine.

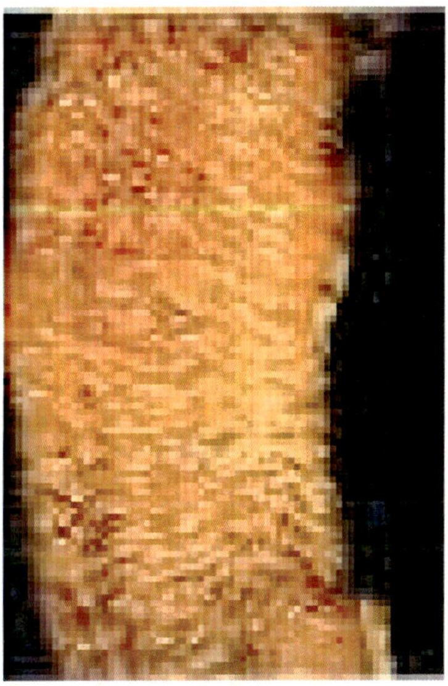

Fig. 5.31: Photograph showing corrugations in large intestine indicative of chronic enteritis

Microscopic features

- Proliferation of fibrous tissue in lamina propria.
- Infiltration of macrophages, lymphocytes, plasma cells.
- Atrophy of intestinal glands.

Necrotic Enteritis

Necrotic enteritis is characterized by necrosis of mucosal epithelium of intestine leading to erosions/ulcer formation and exposition of underlying tissues (Figs. 5.32 to 5.34).

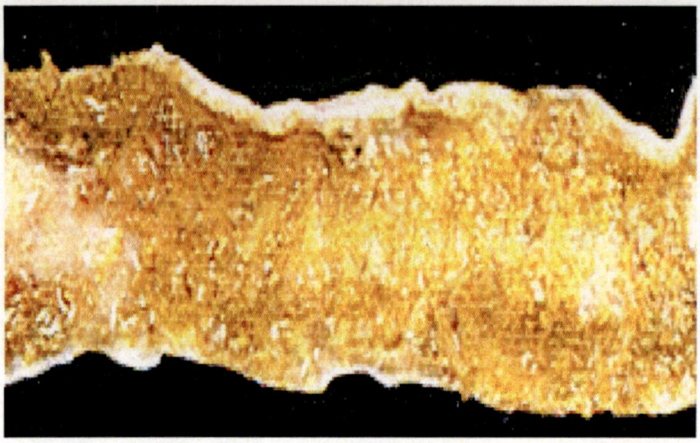

Fig. 5.32: Photograph showing necrotic enteritis in birds due to clostridia

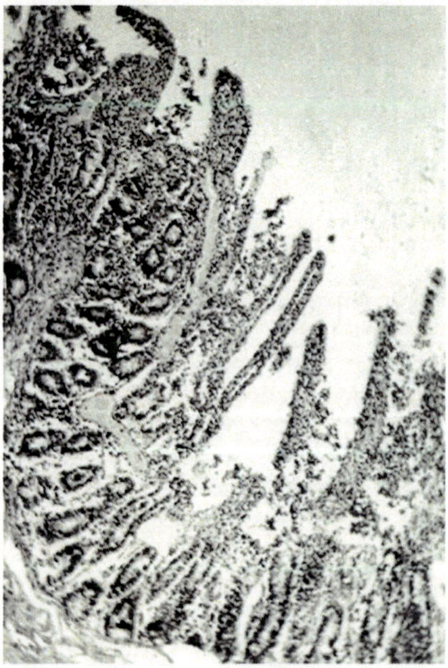

Fig. 5.33: Photograph showing necrotic enteritis

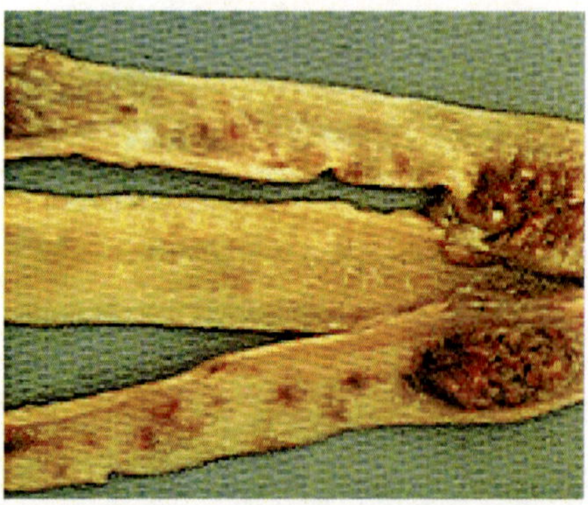

Fig. 5.34: Photomicrograph showing necrotic enteritis

Etiology

- Salmonella.
- Rinderpest, rotavirus, cornovirus, Hog cholera virus.
- Coccidia, Histoplasma.
- Niacin deficiency.
- Clostridium sp. after coccidial infection in birds.

Macroscopic features

- Necrotic patches in intestines.
- Fibrinous deposits over necrotic patches like bran deposits.
- Swelling of mesenteric lymphnodes.
- Ulcers in intestine.

Microscopic features

- Congestion and infiltration of mononuclear cells.
- Necrosis and desquamation of intestinal villus epithelium, leading to exposed underlying tissue.
- Ulcers in mucosa.
- Proliferation of crypt epithelium, presence of abnormal epithelium over villus surface.

Parasitic Enteritis

Parasitic enteritis is caused by parasites and is characterized by catarrhal and/or hemorrhagic exudate in intestine, presence of ova/adult parasite and thickening of the wall of intestine (Figs. 5.35 & 5.36).

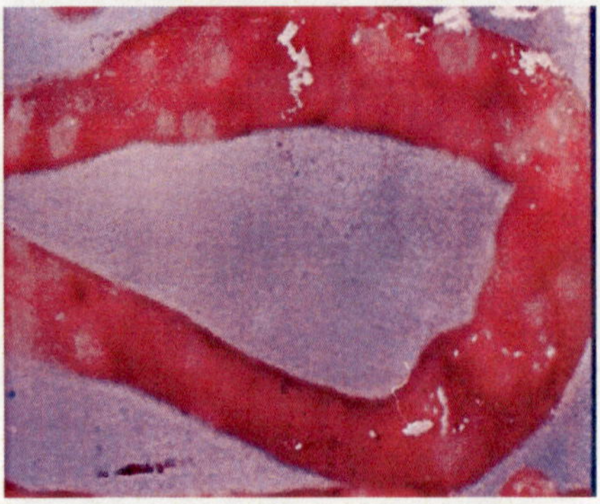

Fig. 5.35: Photograph showing parasitic enteritis (Coccidiosis)

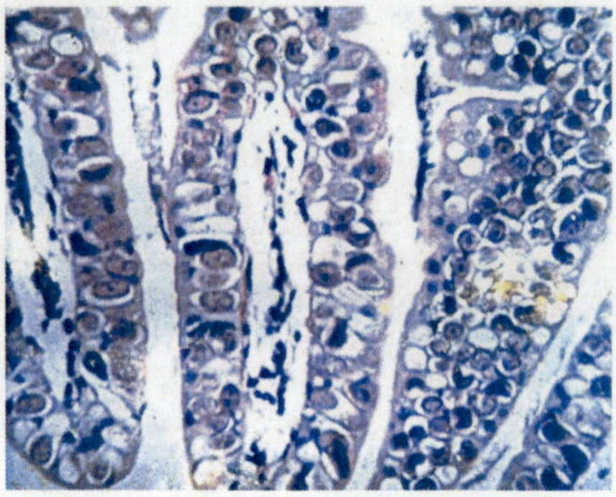

Fig. 5.36: Photomicrograph showing parasitic enteritis (Coccidiosis)

Etiology

- Helminths
- Roundworms
- Tapeworms
- Protozoa
- Coccidia
- Histoplasma

Macroscopic features

- Presence of parasite helminths in the lumen of intestine.
- Thickening of the wall of intestine.
- Catarrhal or hemorrhagic exudate in intestine.

Microscopic features

- Presence of large number of goblet cells in mucosa of intestine.
- Congestion and/or hemorrhage.
- Presence of parasite/ova in the intestinal lumen.
- Infiltration of eosinophils in mucosa and submucosa of the intestines.
- Coccidia can be seen on mucosal scrapings under microscope.

Fibrinous Enteritis

Fibrinous enteritis is the fibrinous inflammation of intestine characterized by presence of fibrinous exudate comprising of pseudomembrane in the mucosa of intestine (Fig. 5.37).

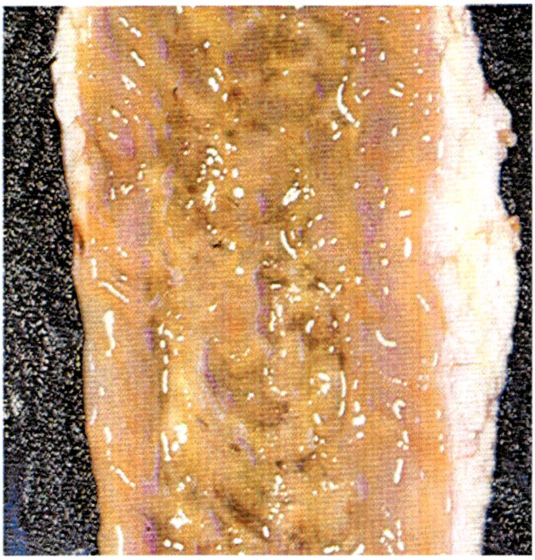

Fig. 5.37: Photograph showing fibrinous enteritis

Etiology

- Salmonella choleraesuis.
- Spherophorus necrophorus.

Macroscopic features

- Presence of diphtheritic membrane over mucosa of intestine.
- Button ulcers.
- Sometimes, diphtheritic membrane covers the faeces.

Microscopic features

- Congestion and hemorrhage in intestine. Thickening of intestinal wall due to fibrinous exudate.
- Fibrin network in mucosa.

Granulomatous Enteritis

Granulomatous enteritis is caused by bacteria or fungi and is characterized by granuloma formation in the intestines (Figs. 5.38 & 5.39).

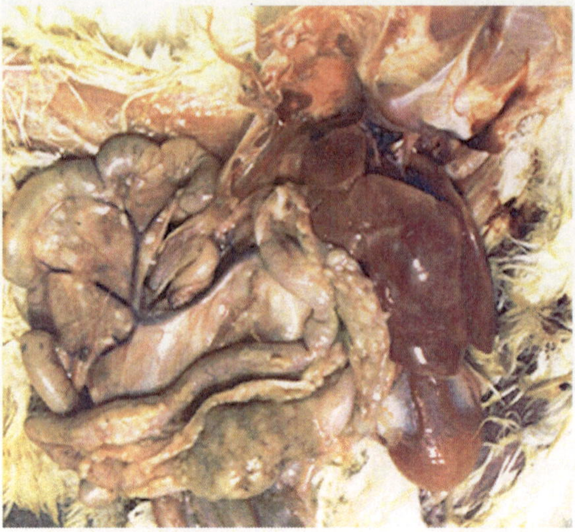

Fig. 5.38: Photograph showing granulomatous lesion in duodenum of poultry

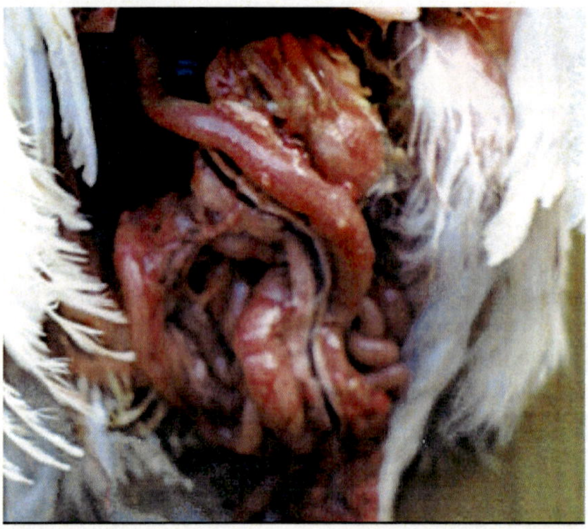

Fig. 5.39: Photograph showing small tiny necrotic granulomatous lesion on intestine

Etiology

- Mycobacterium tuberculosis.
- Coli granuloma – *E. coli* in poultry (Hjarre's disease).
- Coccidioidomycosis / candidiasis.

Macroscopic features

- Granulomatous about cm diameter elevated/ raised areas on the serus surface of intestine.
- Thickening of the wall of intestine.
- Small, tiny, white necrotic nodules on serosa.

Microscopic features

- Granuloma formation consisting of central necrosed area covered by lymphocytes, macrophages, epithelioid cells, giant cells and fibrous connective tissue.
- Extensive proliferation of fibrous tissue.
- Presence of bacteria / fungus in the lesion.

Table 5.1: Differential features of various types of Enteritis

	Catarrhal	Hemorrhagic	Chronic	Necrotic	Parasitic	Fibrinous	Granulomatous
Macroscopic features	1. Presence of catarrhal exudate in lumen of intestine and congestion. 2. Thickening of the wall of intestine. 3. Presence of parasites in lumen of intestine	1.Hemorrhagic exudate in intestines; blood mixed intestinal contents. 2. Petechial or echymotic hemorrhage in mucosa and submucosa of intestine. 3. Presence of erosions/ ulcers in mucosa.	1. Thickening of the wall of intestine (Corrugations in Johne's disease). 2. Thickmucous cover over mucosa of intestine 3.Transverse corrugations in the large intestine. 4.Granulomatous nodules in duodenum. 5. Small, round, raised necrotic foci on serosal surface of intestine covering whole length of intestine.	1. Necrotic patches in intestines. 2. Fibrinous deposits over necrotic patches like bran deposits 3. Swelling of mesenteric lymphnodes 4. Ulcers in intestine.	1. Presence of parasite helminths in the lumen of intestine. 2. Thickening of the wall of intestine. 3. Catarrhal or haemorrhagic exudate in intestine	1.Presence of diphtheritic membrane over mucosa of intestine. 2. Button ulcers 3. Sometimes diphtheritic membrane covers the faeces	1.Granulomatous about one cm diameter elevated/ raised areas on the serus surface of intestine. 2. Thickening of the wall of intestine. 3. Small, tiny, white necrotic nodules on serosa.

	Catarrhal	Hemorrhagic	Chronic	Necrotic	Parasitic	Fibrinous	Granulomatous
Microscopic features	1. Increased number of goblet cells in intestinal villi, reduced length of villi. 2.Congestion 3.Infiltration of polymorpho nuclear and mononuclear cells.	1.Haemorrhage in the mucosa of intestine 2. Infiltration of neutrophils and mononuclear cells. 3. Erosion or ulcers in intestinal mucosa	1. Proliferation of fibrous tissue in lamina propria. 2. Infiltration of macrophages, lymphocytes, plasma cells. 3. Atrophy of intestinal glands.	1. Congestion and infiltration of mononuclear cells. 2. Necrosis and desquamation of intestinal villus epithelium, leading to exposed underlying tissue. 3. Ulcers in mucosa. 4. Proliferation of crypt epithelium, presence of abnormal epithelium over villus surface.	1. Presence of large number of goblet cells in mucosa of intestine. 2. Congestion and/ or haemorrhage. 3. Presence of parasite/ova in the intestinal lumen 4. Infiltration of eosinophils in mucosa and submucosa of the intestines. 5. Coccidia can be seen on mucosal scrapings under microscope.	1.Congestion and haemorrhage in intestine. 2. Thickening of intestinal wall due to fibrinous exudate. 3. Fibrin network in mucosa.	1. Granuloma formation consisting of central necrosed area covered by lymphocytes, macrophages, epithelioid cells, giant cells and fibrous connective tissue 2. Extensive proliferation of fibrus tissue. 3. Presence of bacteria/ fungus in the lesion.

Intestinal Obstruction

Obstruction of intestines may occur as a result of foreign body, enterolith, piliconcretions, phytobezoars, polybezoars or due to hypermotility of intestines leading to intussusception, volvulus or torsion.

Piliconcretions

Piliconcretions are hair balls mostly found in stomach/intestines of animals having habit of licking. This vice is more common in suckling calves and in animals with pica related to phosphorus deficiency. The hairs are accumulated in stomach which become in rounded shape due to movements of stomach and look like balls. Such hair balls are not degradable in gastrointestinal tract and may cause obstruction (Fig. 5.40).

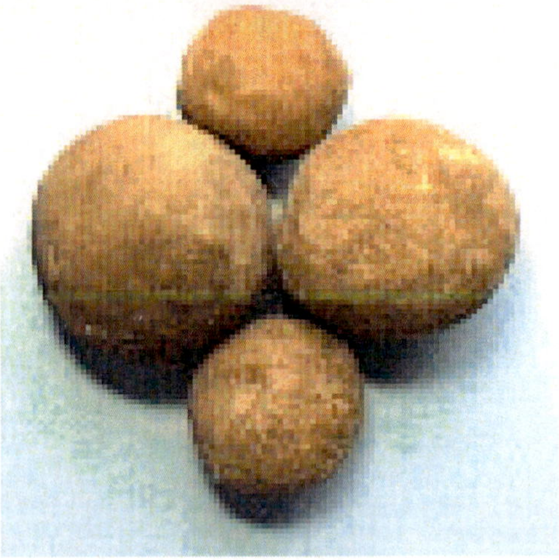

Fig. 5.40: Photograph showing piliconcretions (hair balls) recovered from stomach of calves

Phytobezoars/Polybezoars

Concretions formed in gastrointestinal tract as a result of deposition of salts around a nidus of undigested plants or polythenes. They may cause obstruction in gastrointestinal tract (Fig. 5.41).

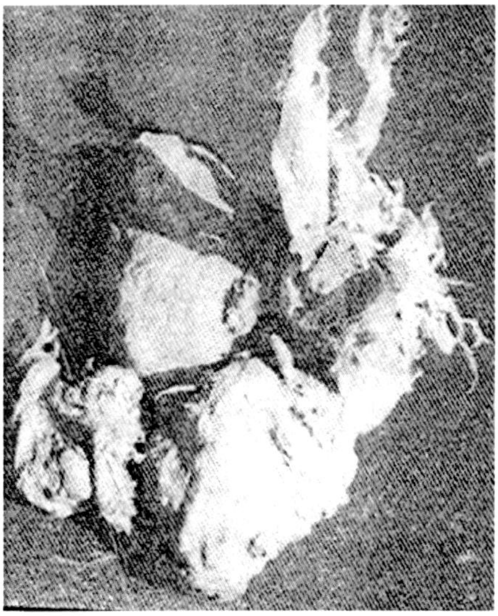

Fig. 5.41: Photograph showingpolybezoars recovered from stomach of a barking deer

Foreign bodies

Foreign bodies like rubber balls, nuts, bones, stones, plastic and rubber materials, polythenes may obstruct the intestinal tract as they are not degradable in the gastrointestinal tract.

Hernia

Hernia is presence of intestinal loop in umbilical area, scrotum or inguinal cavity which causes passive congestion, oedema and obstruction in intestines.

Intussusception

Intussusception is telescoping of intestine means a portion of intestine enters in caudal segment due to violent peristaltic movement. It causes obstruction, passive congestion and oedema (Fig. 5.42).

A

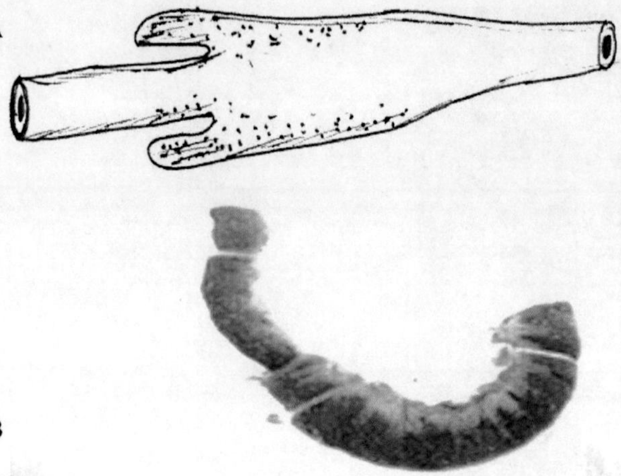

B

Fig. 5.42: Diagram (A) and photograph (B) showing intussusception in intestine

Volvulus

In volvulus, the loop of intestine passes through a tear in mesentry. It causes obstruction at both ends of loop (Fig. 5.43).

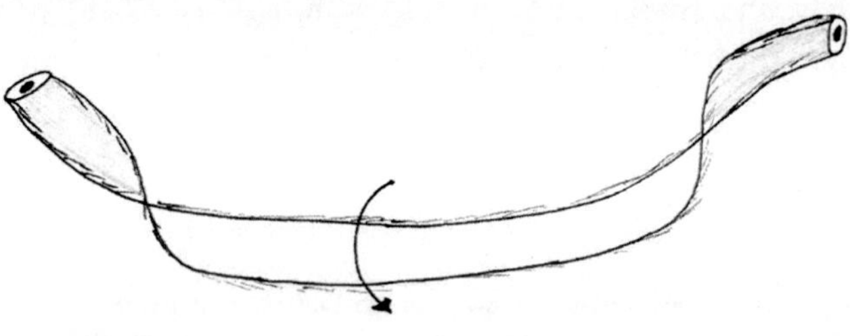

Fig. 5.43: Diagram showing volvulus in intestine

Torsion

Torsion is twisting of intestine upon itself causing obstruction (Fig. 5.44).

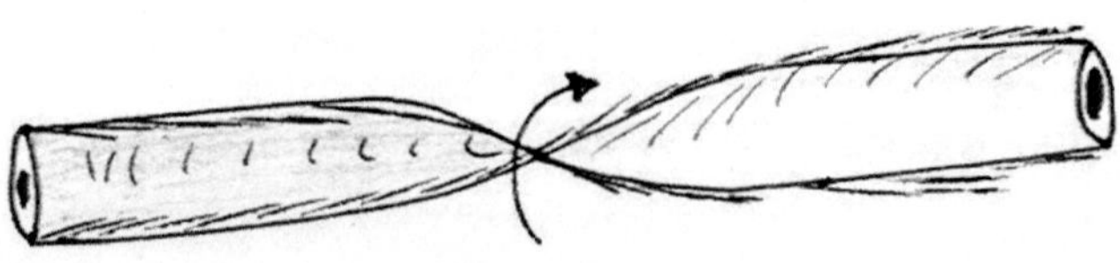

Fig. 5.44: Diagram showing torsion in intestine

Enterolith

Concretions in intestines particularly in horses are responsible for obstruction of intestinal tract and cause "colic in horse" and enterocolitis (Fig. 5.45).

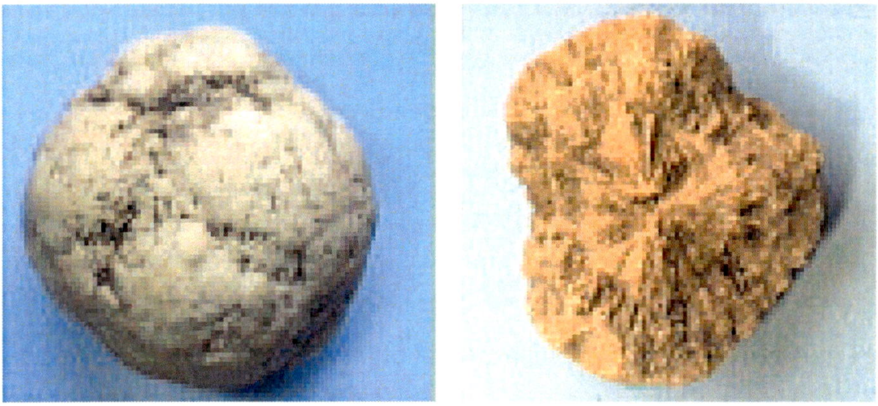

A B

Fig. 5.45: Photograph showing A. enterolith recovered from colon of a horse B. cross section of enterolith showing lamellated deposition of salts

Typhlitis

Typhlitis is the inflammation of caecum. It is particularly important in poultry, caused by protozoan parasites and characterized by hemorrhage, thickening of the wall, presence of cheesy exudates and/or necrotic ulcers (Fig. 5.46).

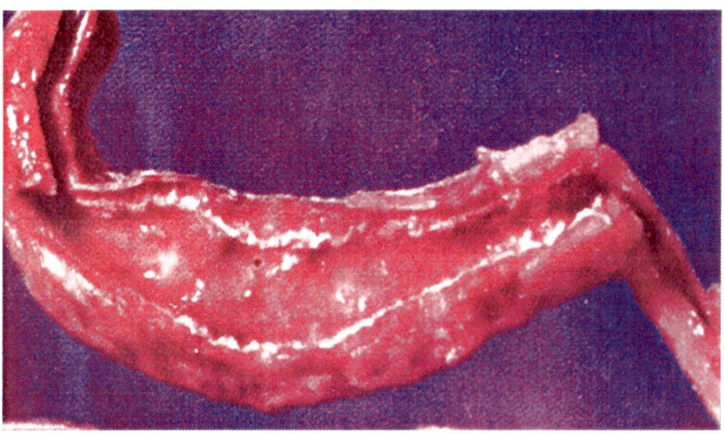

Fig. 5.46: Photograph showing typhlitis in poultry

Etiology

- Eimeria tennella.
- Histomonas meleagridis.

Macroscopic features

- Haemorrhage in caecum, blood mixed contents.
- Thickening of the wall, with congestion and cheesy exudates.

Presence of necrotic ulcers in caecum in case of histomoniasis which is further supported by round, depressed, yellowish-green areas of necrosis in liver.

Microscopic features

- Congestion, haemorrhage, necrosis.
- Presence of protozoan parasites.
- Necrotic hepatic lesions.

Hepatitis

Hepatitis is the inflammation of liver. It may be acute or chronic. Acute hepatitis is characterized by the presence of degeneration and necrosis of hepatocytes and infiltration of neutrophils and mononuclear cells along with hyperemia and/or hemorrhage (Figs. 5.47 to 5.51).

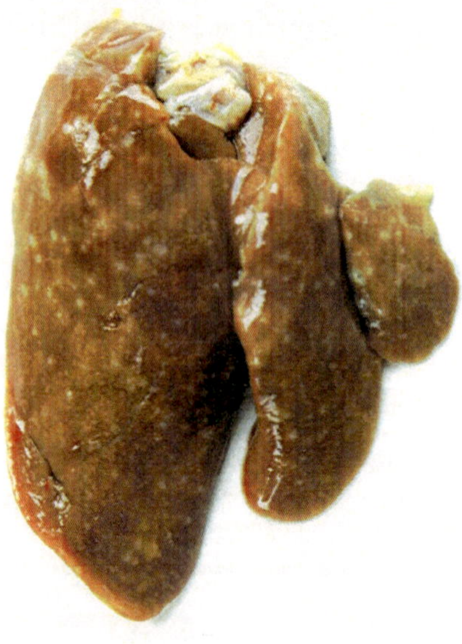

Fig. 5.47: Photograph of liver showing hepatitis

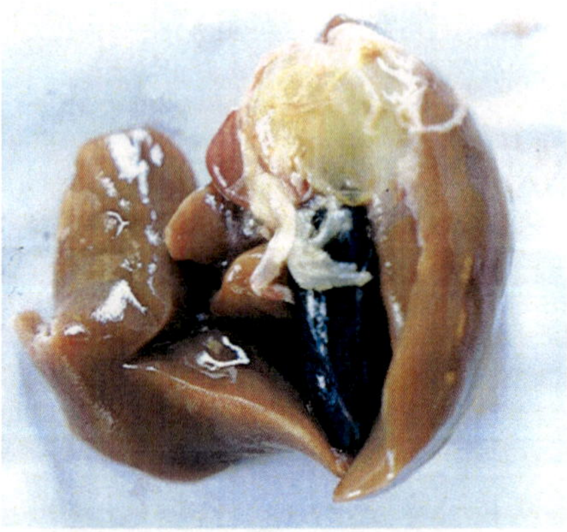

Fig. 5.48: Photograph showing presence of fibrinous membrane on liver (Colisepticemia.) with focal necrosis

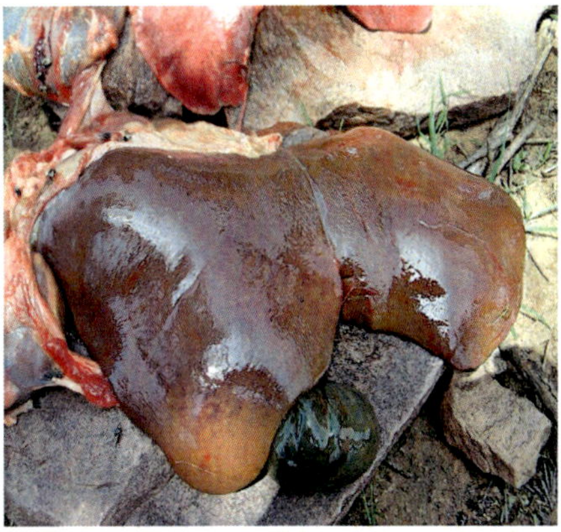

Fig. 5.49: Photograph of liver showing icterus and necrotic lesions

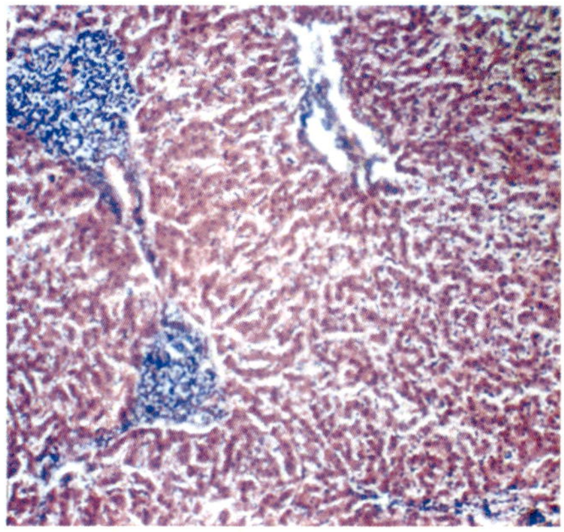

Fig. 5.50: Photomicrograph showing focal necrosis

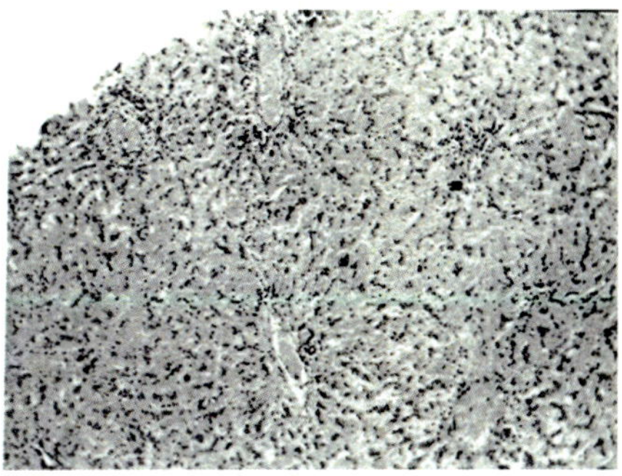

Fig. 5.51: Photomicrograph of liver showing diffuse necrosis

Etiology

- Bacteria – Necrobacillosis, Salmonella, *E. coli.*
- Virus – ICH.
- Chemicals – Carbon tetrachloride.
- Parasites – *Fasciola gigantica, Fasciola hepatica.*
- Plant toxins- Lantana

Macroscopic features

- Enlargement of liver.
- Congestion and/or hemorrhage.
- Presence of necrotic patches in liver.
- Presence of fibrinous diphtheritic membrane on liver.

Microscopic features

- Cloudy swelling and/or fatty changes in liver.
- Congestion in blood vessels and in sinusoidal area.
- Infiltration of neutrophils, macrophages and lymphocytes.
- Necrosis of hepatic parenchyma.

In acute toxic hepatitis there is necrosis of hepatocytes. According to location it can be classified as under which is helpful in making diagnosis.

- Diffused necrosis covers a considerable area crossing over the lobular boundaries.
- Focal necrosis occupying only a part of lobule e.g. EHV induced aborted foetal liver.
- Peripheral necrosis is characterized by necrosis at the periphery of lobule which occurs due to presence of strong toxins in blood.
- Midzonal necrosis have necrosis of cells in midway of periphery and centre of lobule.
- Centrilobular necrosis is characterized by necrosis of hepatocytes around the central vein and occurs due to stagnation of blood with toxaemia.
- Paracentral necrosis is characterized by necrosis of hepatocytes at one side of central vein e.g. Rift valley fever.

Cirrhosis

Cirrhosis is the chronic inflammation of liver characterized by extensive fibrosis, hepatic degeneration and necrosis (Fig. 5.52 to 5.54).

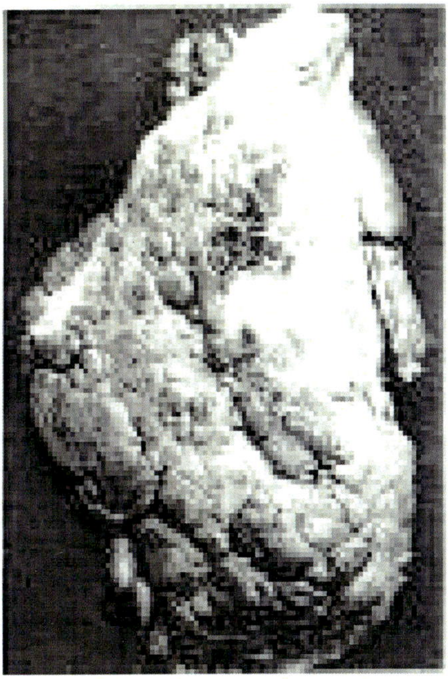

Fig. 5.52: Photograph showing cirrhosis in liver

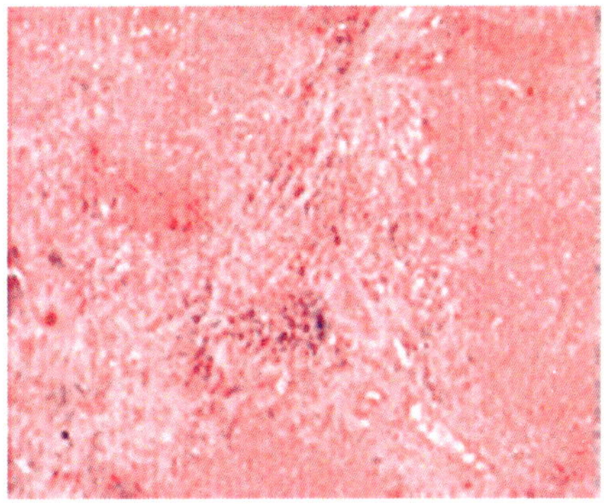

Fig. 5.53: Photomicrograph showing cirrhosis in liver

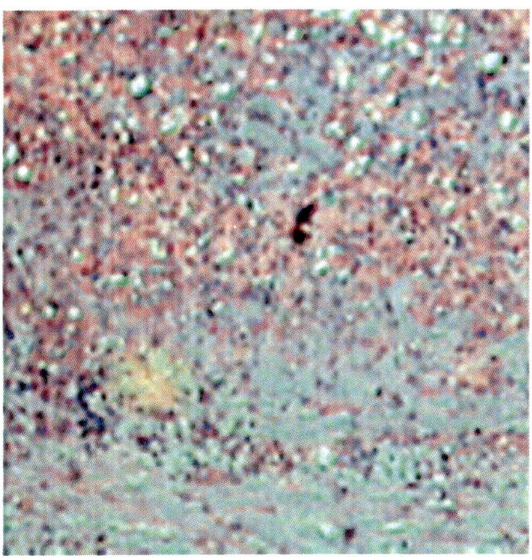

Fig. 5.54: Photomicrograph showing cirrhosis in liver

Etiology

- Bacteria – Salmonella, *Spherophorus necrophorous*.

- Virus – Infectious canine hepatitis.
- Chemicals – Carbon tetrachloride.
- Parasites – *Fasciola hepatica, F. giantica.*
- Poisons/toxins – Aflatoxins.
- Once cirrhosis of liver starts, it is not checked even after removal of the cause as the newly formed fibrous tissue itself acts as an irritant to cause further proliferation of fibroblasts.

Macroscopic features

- Liver becomes hard and firm.
- Surface of liver becomes uneven and nodular.
- Size of liver becomes reduced due to atrophy.
- Colour becomes yellowish, grey.

Microscopic features

- Increase in fibrous tissue within and around lobules.
- Infiltration of macrophages and lymphocytes.
- Central vein is either absent or placed eccentrically.
- Hepatocytes show degenerative and necrotic changes. Biliary cirrhosis is characterized by proliferation of fibrous tissue around the bile ducts encircling them e.g. Fasciola giantica.
- Glissonian cirrhosis is mostly confined to areas at a short distance beneath the capsule.
- Pigment cirrhosis is associated with yellow discolouration.
- Central or cardiac cirrhosis is increase in fibrous tissue around the central vein as a result of chronic passive congestion.
- Parasitic cirrhosis occurs due to damage caused by migration of parasites e.g. Ascaris lumbricoides, Schistosoma sp.

Cholecystitis

Cholecystitis is the inflammation of gall bladder characterized by congestion, thickening of wall and infiltration of mononuclear cells. Cholangitis is the inflammation of bile duct (Figs. 5.55 & 5.56).

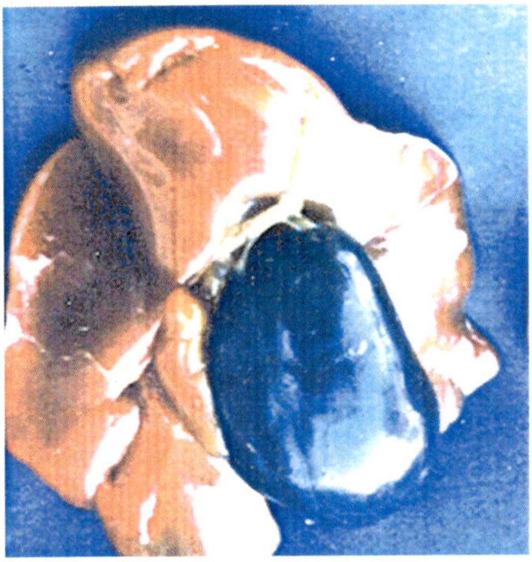

Fig. 5.55: Photograph showing cholecystitis in birds

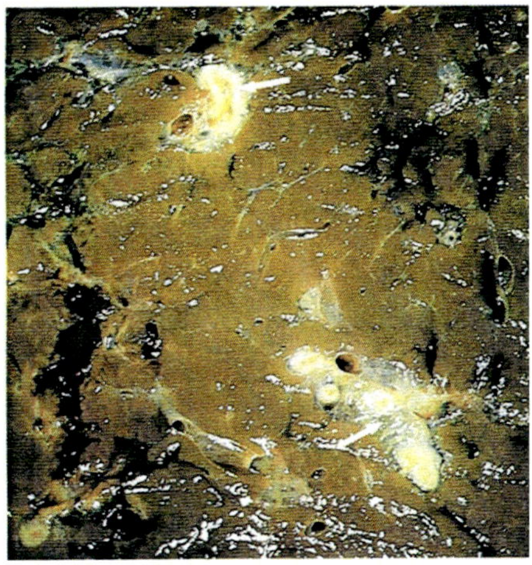

Fig. 5.56: Photograph showing cholangitis

Etiology

- Parasites – *Fasciola* sp.
- Foreign body – Stones
- Bacteria – *E. coli*.

Macroscopic features

- Thickening of the wall of gall bladder.
- On opening of gall bladder, there may be parasites/stones/foreign body.
- Contents of gall bladder may be watery or thick oily.

Microscopic features

- Congestion.
- Proliferation of fibrous tissue in the wall of gall bladder.
- Infiltration of mononuclear cells.
- Increased number of mucus secreting cells.

Pancreatitis

Pancreatitis is the inflammation of pancreas characterized by necrosis of pancreatic tissue, infiltration of neutrophils and mononuclear cells and fibrous tissue proliferation.

Etiology

- Bacteria.
- Virus- Reovirus in poultry.
- Parasites.

Macroscopic features

- Pancreas becomes pale, swollen, oedematous.
- In chronic cases, atrophy of pancreas.
- Pancreas becomes hard, firm, and fibrous.

Microscopic features

- Necrosis of pancreatic cells.
- Oedema, infiltration of leucocytes, hemorrhage.
- Fibrosis characterized by proliferation of fibroblasts.

Pathology of Peritonium

Peritonitis is the inflammation of peritoneum characterized by hemorrhagic suppurative, serofibrinous or nodular lesions (FIg. 5.57 & 5.58).

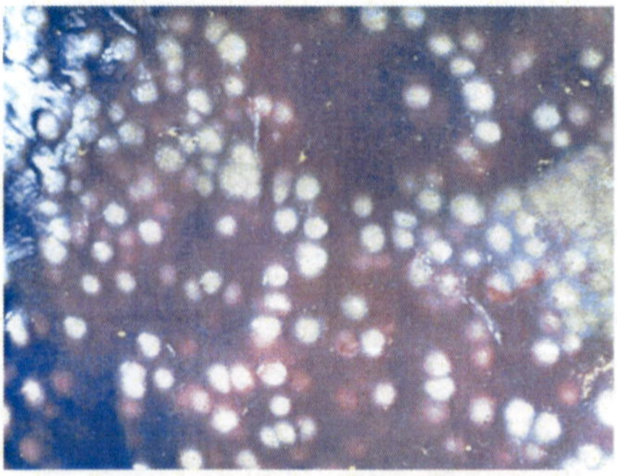

Fig. 5.57: Photograph showing pearly disease

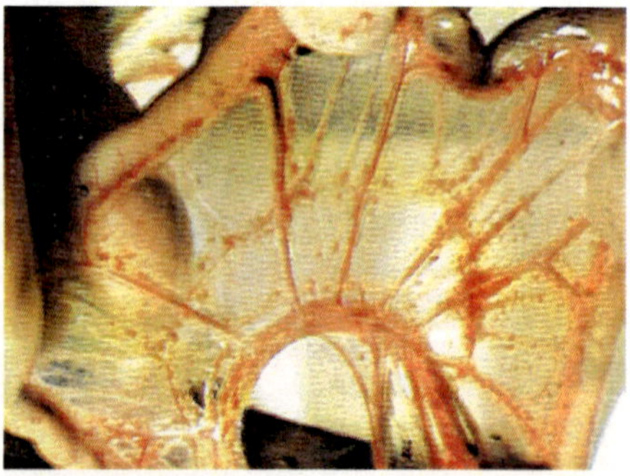

Fig. 5.58: Photograph showing haemorrhage in mesentery due to peritonitis

Etiology

- Bacteria – Staphylococci, *Mycobacterium* sp.
- Virus.
- Neoplasia.
- Parasites .

Macroscopic features

- Serofibrinous, fibrinous, hemorrhagic, suppurative or granulomatous lesions.
- Accumulation of clear fluid

Hydroperitoneum or Ascites.

- Presence of nodules in tuberculosis is also termed as "***Pearly disease***".

Microscopic features

- Serofibrinous, suppurative or granulomatous lesions.
- Thickening of peritoneum, adhesions due to fibrosis.

6

Pathology of Hemopoitic and Immune System

Developmental Anomalies

Hereditary anemia

Hereditary anemia has been reported in mice due to defects in erythropoiesis or reduced vitality of erythrocytes. Erythropenia along with leucopenia occurs in mouse foetus on 20th day of gestation due to defective autosomal chromosome 4. Sex linked anemia in mouse is hypochromic with deficient bone marrow and occurs in hemizygus males or homozygus females. This anemia occurs due to deficiency of iron as a result of poor absorption from gastrointestinal tract.

Autoimmune hemolytic anemia in foals

It occurs due to incompatible blood group antigens of male and female parents. The mare does not have that blood group antigen but foetus acquires it from father. The foetal blood exposed to dam through placental exchanges leads to induction of antibody production in mares against foetal blood group antigen. These antibodies accumulate in colustrum and when foal suck the milk from mares, they are readily absorbed through G.I. tract of foals in blood and cause destruction of erythrocytes leading to anemia.

Congenital defects in lymphocytes

Congenital defects in lymphocytes are classified under stem cell aplasia/agenesis leading to combined immunodeficiency with absence of both T- and B-lymphocytes in Arabian foals. It occurs either due to inherited gene defect or differentiation/ maturation defects in lymphocytes. It is characterized by agammaglobulinemia, lymphopenia, hypoplasia of thymus, lymphnodes and spleen.

Chediak-Higashi Syndrome

This syndrome is related with defects in phagocytic cells such as defective neutrophils and monocytes. The defects are in chemotaxis, engulfment and killing of bacteria and associated with defective assembly of cytoplasmic microtubules responsible for degranulation and release of lysosomal enzymes, there is depression of superoxide anions leading to persistent bacterial infections.

Anemia

Anemia is the decrease in number of erythrocytes or hemoglobin concentration in erythrocytes per unit of blood and is characterized by pale mucus membrane, dyspnoea, cardiac hypertrophy and weakness. Anemia is classified according to morphological characteristics of erythrocytes and on the basis of causative factors. Morphologically, anemia is classified as macrocytic, normocytic and microcytic depending on the size of red blood cells and normochromic and hypochromic based on the presence of quantity of hemoglobin in RBC. Macrocytic anemia is characterized by increased size of RBC and occurs due to acute blood loss or hemolysis resulting in excessive production and availability of immature erythrocytes in blood. Such cells also have reduced amount of hemoglobin and are termed as hypochromic.

Macrocytic normochromic anemia is increase size of RBC with normal hemoglobin and has been observed in deficiency of folic acid, niacin and vitamin B_{12}. Normocytic anemia is most common in animals occurs due to neoplasia, irradiation and is also known as aplastic anemia as a result of aplasia or agenesis of RBC. In Normocytic normochromic, normal size of RBC with normal hemoglobin occurs as a result of depression of erythrogenesis. Microcytic anemia is reduction in size of erythrocytes with decreased hemoglobin (Microcytic hypochromic) and occurs in deficiency of iron and pyridoxine or chronic blood loss.

In anemia, the size of RBC varies markedly, some being of large size and some of small size and is known as anisocytosis. The presence of abnormal shape (elongated, angular, ovoid, distorted) of RBC is termed as poikilocytosis. In some blood smears, there are nucleated RBC's which are immature due to increased production to meet the demand. Sometimes, the erythrocytes have minute dark spots known as basophilic stippling which occurs in acute blood loss. Some erythrocytes stain unevenly with some dark and light colour spots and are known as polychromatophilia which is an indication of active erythrogenesis. The denaturation and precipitation of hemoglobin leads to appearance of purplish granules in RBC near the cytoplasmic membrane which are known as "Heinz bodies". According to etiological factors, anemia is classified as hemolytic, haemorrhagic or deficiency anemia.

Hemolytic Anemia

Hemolytic anemia occurs due to excessive lysis of erythrocytes and is characterized by icterus, hemoglobinuria and presence of nucleated erythrocytes in blood and hemosiderosis in spleen.

Etiology

- Infections e.g. *Anaplasma* spp. Babesia spp., Equine infectious anemia virus.
- Toxins/ poisons e.g. snake venom, chronic lead poisoning.
- Immune mechanisms e.g. autoimmunity against erythrocytes (Fig. 6.1).

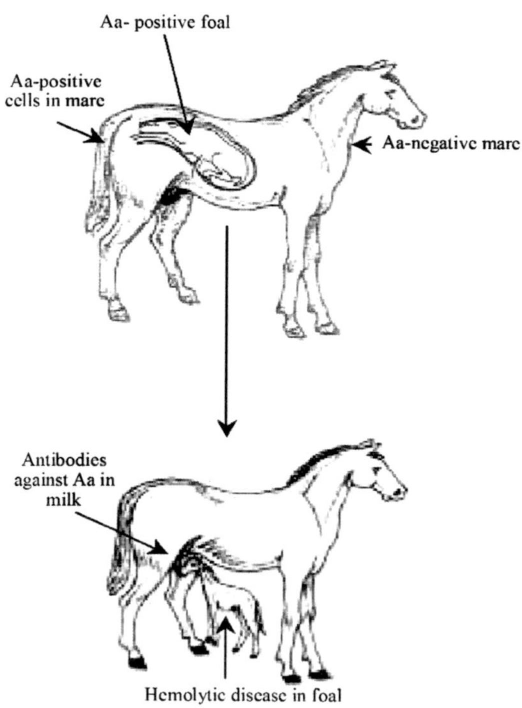

Fig. 6.1: Diagram showing autoimmune hemolytic anemia in foals

Macroscopic features

- Pale mucus membranes.
- Icterus.
- Blood is thin, watery.
- Hemoglobinurea.

Microscopic features

- Decreased number of erythrocytes.
- Presence of nucleated/immature RBC in blood.
- Hemosiderin laden cells in spleen.

Hemorrhagic Anemia

Hemorrhagic anemia occurs due to severe hemorrhage, extravasation of blood and is characterized by pale mucus membrane and hemorrhage in body.

Etiology

- Infections e.g. Acute septicemic diseases.
- Toxins/poisons e.g. Bracken fern poisoning.
- Parasites e.g. *Hemonchus contortus*.
- Deficiency e.g. vitamin C deficiency.

Macroscopic features

- Petechiae or echymotic hemorrhage.
- Pale mucus membrane.
- Hematuria.

Microscopic features

- Hemorrhage in various tissues /organs.
- Macrocytic or normocytic characters of RBC.
- Poikilocytosis.
- Hyperplasia of bone marrow.

Deficiency Anemia

Deficiency anemia occurs as a result of deficiency of iron, copper, cobalt and vitamins and is characterized by pale mucus membrane, weak and debilitated body and decreased number of erythrocytes with hypochromasia in blood.

Etiology

- Deficiency of iron.
- Deficiency of copper.

- Deficiency of cobalt.
- Deficiency of vitamin B_{12}, Pyridoxine, riboflavin and folic acid.
- Parasitic infestation may lead to deficiency.

Macroscopic features

- Pale mucus membrane.
- Thin watery blood with light red colour.
- Weak and debilitated carcass.
- Heavy parasitic load in gastrointestinal tract.

Microscopic features

- Microcytic hypochromic erythrocytes.
- Poikilocytosis.

Toxic Aplastic Anemia

Toxic aplastic anemia is agenesis or aplasia of hemopoietic tissues in bone marrow and there is lack of erythrocyte production. It is characterized by the absence of developmental stages of erythrocytes viz., normoblasts, megaloblasts etc.

Etiology

- Radiation e.g. X-rays, γ rays, or UV rays.
- Sulfonamides.
- Bracken fern toxicity.
- Uremia.
- Feline panleukopenia.

Macroscopic features

- Pale mucus membrane.
- Weak and debilitated animal.
- Dyspnoea.
- Bone marrow becomes yellow/fatty (Fig. 6.2).

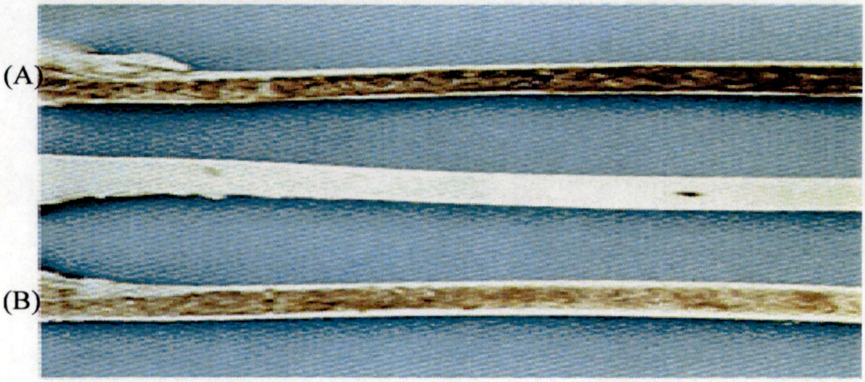

Fig. 6.2: Photograph showing toxic aplastic anemia (A). Normal (B). Yellow bone marrow

Microscopic features

- Absence of developmental stages or RBC such as normoblasts, megaloblasts etc.
- Agranulocytosis i.e. reduction of WBC in circulating blood.
- Bone marrow becomes fatty.

Autoimmune Hemolytic Anemia

Autoimmune hemolytic anemia occurs as a result of destruction of erythrocytes by immune mechanisms developed against erythrocytes.

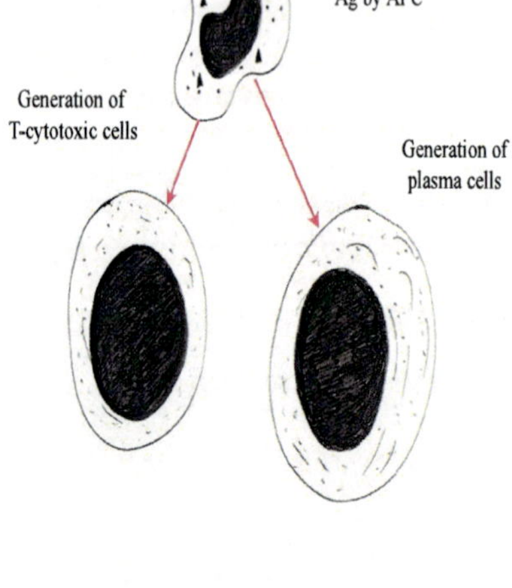

Etiology

- Autoimmune hemolytic anemia in foals.
- Antibodies produced against own RBC of an animal (Fig. 6 .3).
- Equine infectious anemia.
- Anaplasmosis.
- Systemic lupus erythematosus.

Table 6.1: Differential features of various types of Anaemia

	Hemolytic	**Haemorrhagic**	**Deficiency**	**Toxic/ Aplastic**	**Autoimmune Hemolytic**
Macroscopic features	1. Pale mucus Membranes 2. Icterus 3. Blood is thin, watery. 4. Hemoglobinurea	1. Petechiae or Echymotic haemorrhage 2. Pale mucus membrane 3. Hematuria	1. Pale mucus Membrane 2. Thin watery blood with light red colour 3. Weak and debilitated carcass 4. Heavy parasitic load in Gastrointestinal tract.	1. Pale mucus Membrane 2. Weak and debilitated animal 3. Dyspnoea 4. Bone marrow Becomes yellow/ fatty	1. Pale mucus Membrane 2. Enlargement of liver, spleen and Lymphnodes 3. Hemoglobinuria 4. Lameness due to Rheumatoid Arthritis
Microscopic features	1. Decreased number of Erythrocytes 2. Presence of nucleated/ immaturee RBC in blood 3. Hemosiderin laden cells in Spleen	1. Haemorrhage in various tissues / organs 2. Macrocytic or normocytic characters of RBC 3. Poikilocytosis 4. Hyperplasia of bone marrow	1. Microcytic Hypochromic erythrocytes. 2. Poikilocytosis	1. Absence of Developmental stages or RBC such as normoblasts, megaloblasts etc. 2. Agranulocytosis i.e. Reduction of WBC in circulating blood. 3. Bone marrow becomes fatty.	1. Erythrophagocytos is 2. Demonstration of antibodies against own RBC in sera of animals. 3. Active Erythropoiesis 4. Glomerulonephritis

Macroscopic features

- Pale mucus membrane.
- Enlargement of liver, spleen and lymphnodes.
- Hemoglobinuria.
- Lameness due to rheumatoid arthritis. Erythroid leukemia.

Microscopic features

- Erythrophagocytosis.
- Demonstration of antibodies against own RBC in sera of animals.
- Active erythropoiesis.
- Glomerulonephritis.

Polycythemia

Polycythemia is increase in number of erythrocytes in circulating blood. It may be relative increase as a result of dehydration or decrease in plasma volume or absolute due to anoxia.

Etiology

- Dehydration due to diarrhoea, vomiting and loss of fluid in oedema/ inflammation.
- Anoxia in high altitudes.
- Heart diseases e.g. patent ductus arteriosus.
- Severe pulmonary emphysema.

Macroscopic features

- Dehydration, mucus membrane dry, sticky.
- Pulmonary emphysema, fibrosis in lungs.
- Increase hemoglobin concentration.

Microscopic features

- Increased number of erythrocytes
- Severe damage in lungs, congestion, emphysema, fibrosis

Leucocytosis

Leucocytosis is increase in number of leucocytes in circulating blood caused by various infections. There is also increase in white blood cells in blood due to neoplastic condition and is known as Leukemia. As the leucocytes consist of neutrophils, lymphocytes eosinophils, monocytes and basophils; the increase in number of neutrophils is termed as neutrophilia, eosinophils as eosinophilia, lymphocytes as lymphocytosis, basophils as basophilia and of monocytes as monocytosis.

Etiology

- Infections.
- Bacterial infection – neutrophilia.
- Viral infections and chronic bacterial infections – lymphocytosis.
- Parasites – eosinophilia.
- Allergies – basophilia, lymphocytosis.

Macroscopic features

- No characteristic lesion.
- Reactive lymph node hyperplasia.
- Enlargement of lymphoid organs such as spleen, thymus and bursa.

Microscopic features

- Increase in number of total leucocytes in blood.
- Increase in absolute lymphocyte, absolute neutrophil, absolute eosinophil counts.
- Hyperplastic lesions in lymphoid organs.

Leucopenia

Leucopenia is decrease in number of white blood cells. The leucocytes are neutrophils, lymphocytes monocytes, eosinophils and basophils. If there is decrease in number of all 5 cells of leucocytes, it is known as panleucopenia. The decrease in number of neutrophils is termed as neutropenia and lymphocytes as lymphopenia.

Etiology

- Congenital e.g. Chediak-Higashi Syndrome.
- Infections e.g. Feline panleucopenia virus, infectious bursal disease virus.
- Chemicals e.g. Pesticides, heavy metals.
- Radiation e.g. X-rays.

Macroscopic features

- Atrophy of lymphoid organs.
- Recurrent infections, vaccination failures, pyogenic disorders.
- Oedema, haemorrhage in bursa, atrophy of bursa due to fibrosis in IBD infection.

Microscopic features

- Decrease in total leucocyte count and absolute neutrophil and absolute lymphocyte counts.
- Degeneration and necrosis of lymphoid cells in follicles of lymphoid organ.
- Oedema, necrosis, proliferation of fibrous tissue in bursa in IBD infection.

Pathology of Spleen

Splenitis

Splenitis is the inflammation of spleen characterized by enlargement, infiltration of inflammatory cells, proliferation of lymphoid follicles, congestion and oedema followed by proliferation of fibrous tissue (Figs. 6.4 to 6.6).

A **B** **C** **D**

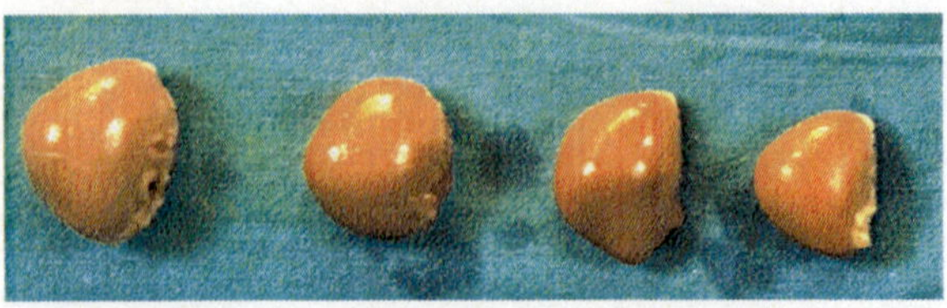

Fig. 6.4: Photograph showing atrophy in spleen
A. Normal, **B, C** and **D** Progressive atrophied of spleen

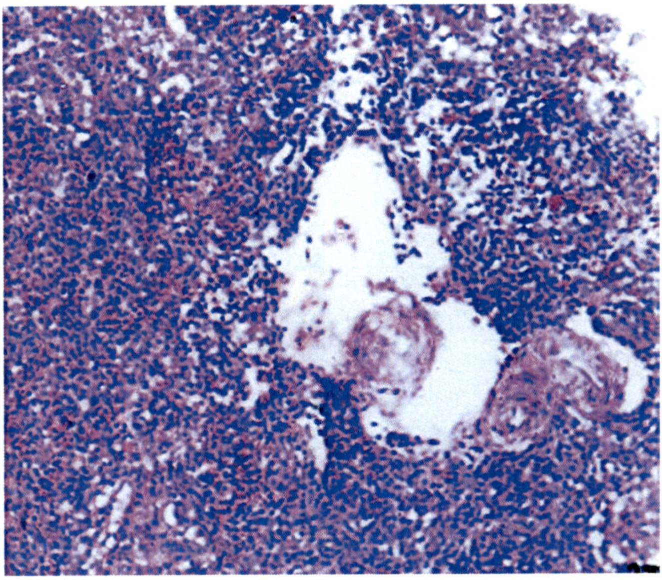

Fig. 6.5: Photomicrograph showing depletion of lymphoid tissue

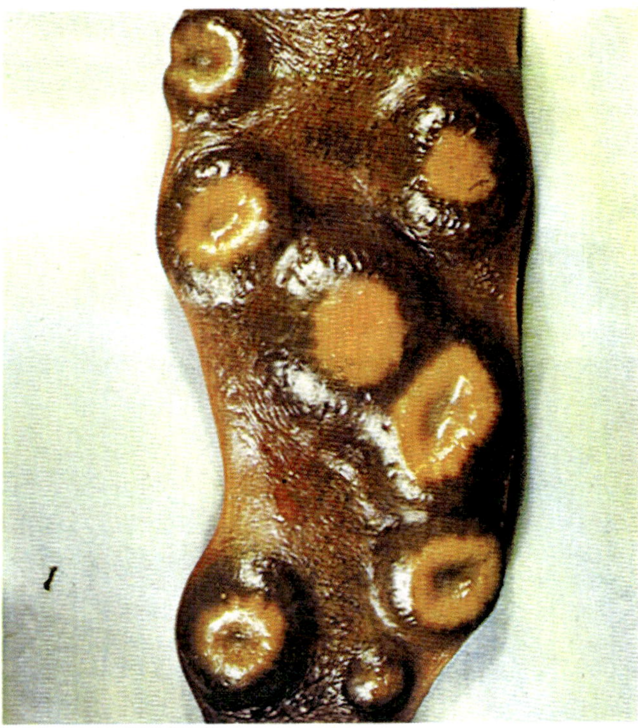

Fig. 6.6: Photograph of spleen showing tubercles/granulomatous lesions

Etiology

- Infections e.g. bacteria, virus.
- Deficiency of vitamins and minerals.
- Amyloidosis.
- Immunodeficiency e.g. environmental pollution

Macroscopic features

- Enlargement of spleen.
- Necrotic patches on spleen.
- In chronic cases or in immunological disorders.
- There is atrophy of spleen due to fibrosis.
- Necrotic patches and congestion leading to mottling.

Microscopic features

- Congestion in spleen.
- Proliferation of lymphoid follicles/cells.
- Oedema.
- In atrophied spleen, proliferation of fibrous tissue, depletion of lymphoid cells/follicles.

Pathology of Lymphnodes

Lymphadenitis

Lymphadenitis is the inflammation of lymphnodes characterized by enlargement/atrophy, congestion proliferation of lymphoid cells/depletion of lymphoid cells, oedema and fibrosis of lymph nodes (Figs. 6.7 to 6.11).

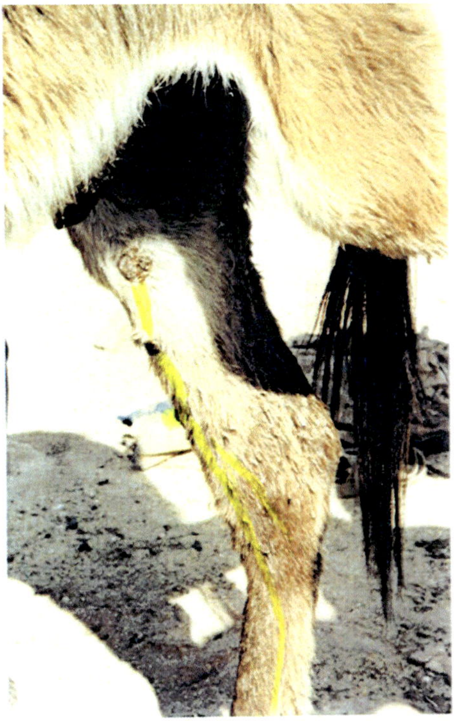

Fig. 6.7: Photograph showing lymphadenitis in horse due to glanders

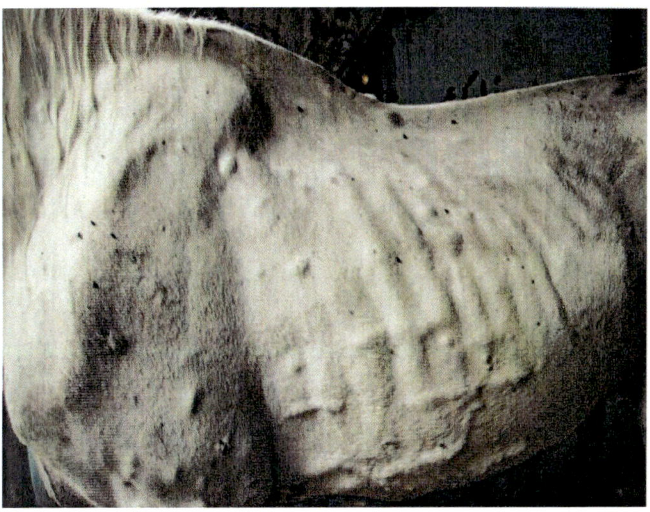

Fig. 6.8: Photograph of horse showing lymphadenitis (Enlargement of lymphnodes, glanders)

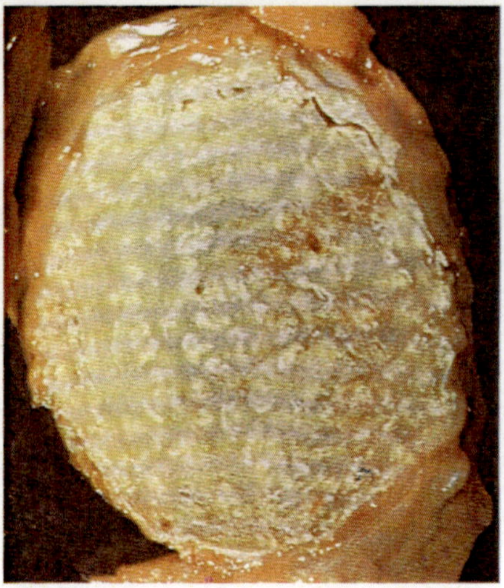

Fig. 6.9: Photograph showing caseous lymphadenitis

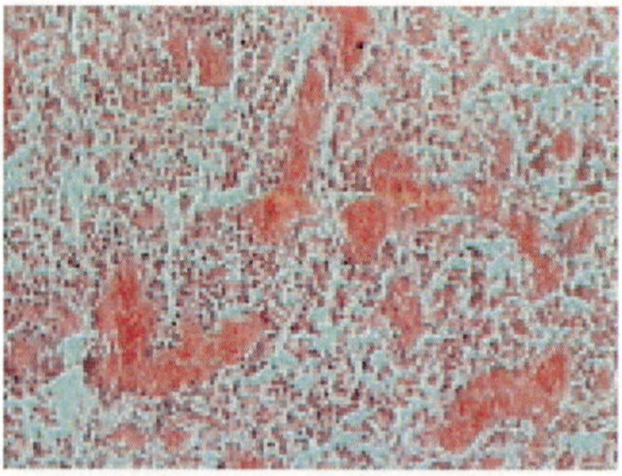

Fig. 6.10: Photomicrograph showing acute lymphadenitis

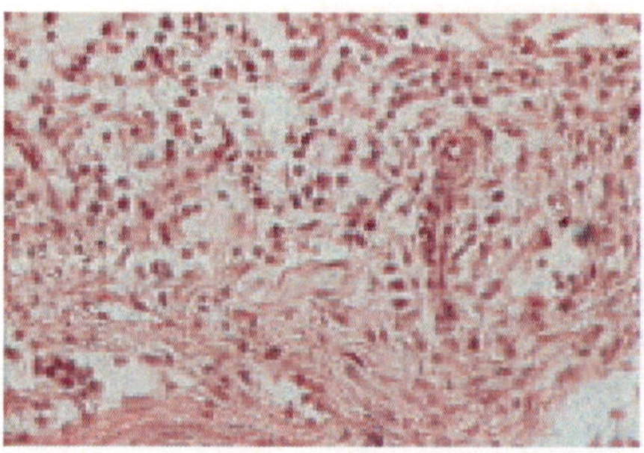

Fig. 6.11: Photomicrograph showing chronic lymphadenitis

Etiology

- Infections e.g. Rinderpest.
- Immunological disorders e.g. immuno-deficiency.
- Deficiency e.g. deficiency of protein.
- Environmental pollution e.g. pesticides, heavy metals.
- Tumors/neoplasm e.g. lymphosarcoma.

Macroscopic features

- Enlargement of lymphnodes.
- Congestion.
- Oedema.
- In chronic cases- fibrosis.
- Atrophy.

Microscopic features

- Congestion, oedema, proliferation of lymphoid cells.
- In chronic cases, proliferation of fibrous tissue, depletion of lymphoid cells.

Pathology of Thymus

Thymoma /Thymic Hyperplasia

It is characterized by congestion and hyperplasia of lymphoid cells in thymus. The inflammation of thymus in chronic cases is characterized by atrophy and proliferation of fibrous tissue (Figs. 6.12 & 6.13).

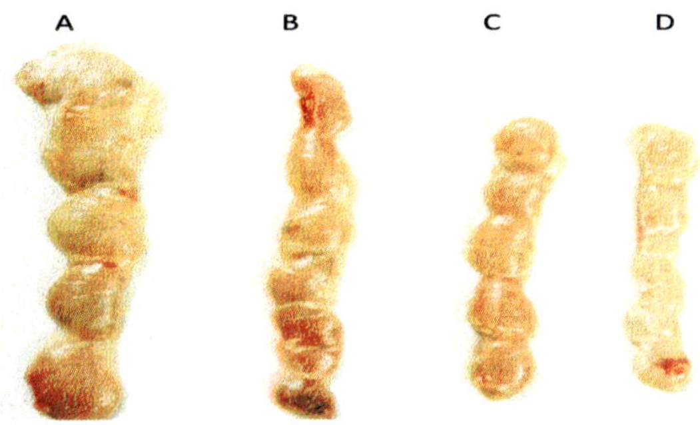

Fig. 6.12: Photograph showing atrophy of thymus A. Normal B, C and D. progressive atrophy

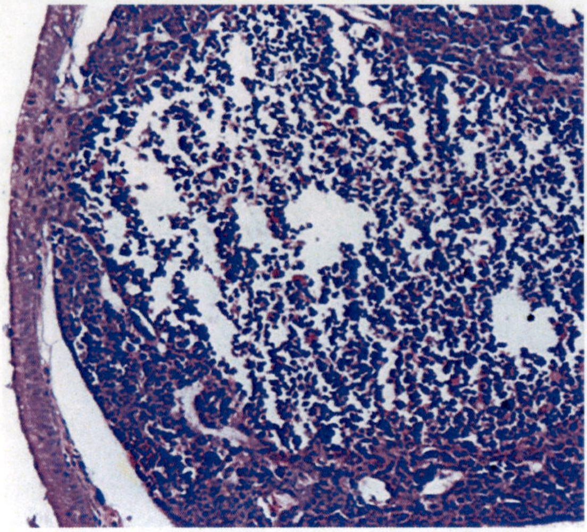

Fig. 6.13: Photomicrograph of thymus showing depletion of lymphoid tissue.

Etiology

Immunological disorders.

Environmental pollution e.g. pesticide, heavy metals.

Toxins/poisons.

Aging e.g. in adult poultry thymus regresses.

Macroscopic features

Congestion, reddening of thymus. Oedema.

Increase in size.

Atrophy, thinning like thread.

Microscopic features

Congestion, oedema.

Proliferation of lymphoid cells. Depletion of lymphoid cells. Proliferation of fibrous tissue.

Pathology of Bursa

Bursitis

Bursitis is the inflammation of bursa of Fabricius in poultry characterized by oedema, congestion, hemorrhage or atrophy and depletion of lymphoid cells (Figs. 6.14 to 6.17).

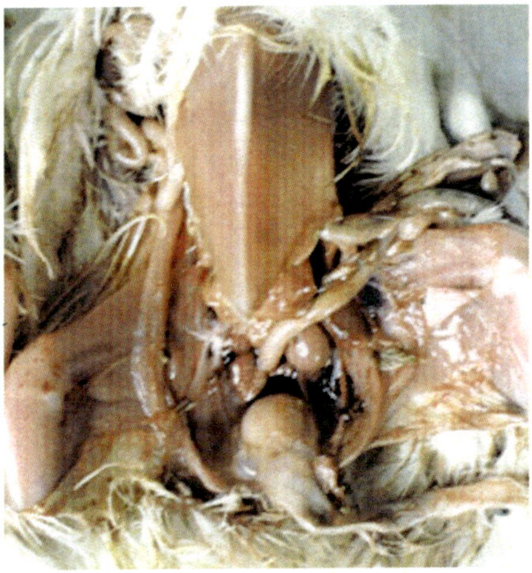

Fig. 6.14: Photograph showing oedema in bursa of Fabricius due to Gumboro disease.

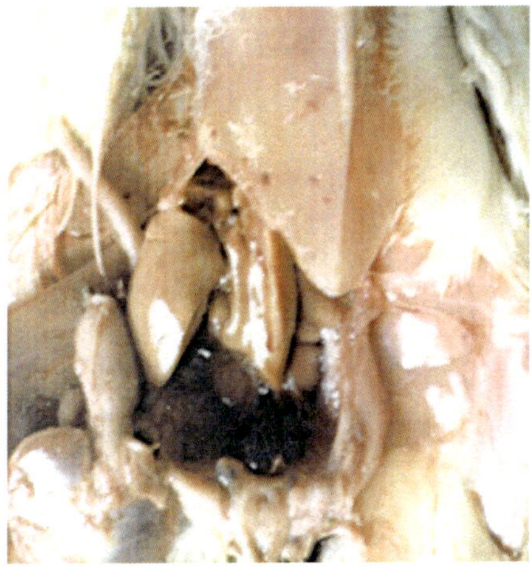

Fig.6.15: Photograph showing haemorrhage in bursa of Fabricius due to Gumboro disease

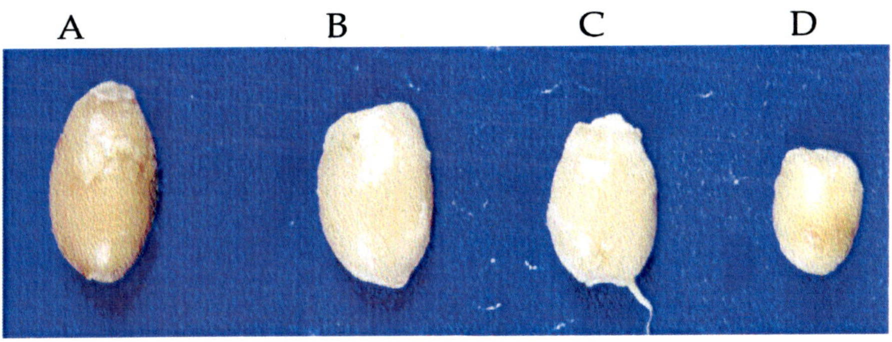

Fig. 6.16: Photograph of bursa of Fabricius showing atrophy and fibrosis (**A**. Normal, **B,C** and **D.** progressive atrophic changes)

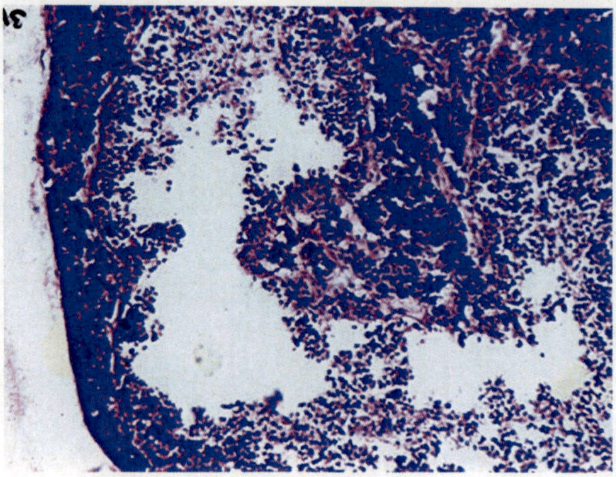

Fig. 6.17: Photomicrograph of bursa of Fabricius showing depletion of lymphoid tissue

Etiology

- Infectious Bursal disease virus (Birnavirus).
- Environmental pollution e.g. Pesticides, heavy metals.

Macroscopic features

- Enlargement of bursa.
- Congestion and/or hemorrhage.
- Oedema.
- In chronic cases, atrophy and fibrosis.

Microscopic features

- Oedema.
- Depletion of lymphoid tissue.
- Degeneration and necrosis of lymphoid cells.
- Congestion and/or hemorrhage.
- Proliferation fibrous tissue.

7

Pathology of Urinary System

Developmental Anomalies

Aplasia

Absence of one or both kidneys. Absence of one kidney is observed in animals with compensatory hypertrophy of another kidney and such animals may survive well.

Hypoplasia

The size of kidneys remains small as they don't grow properly due to defect in a single recessive autosomal gene.

Cyst in kidney

Single or multiple cysts in pig and dog kidney are reported with tinged yellow colour. They may arise from nephron due to its distension. Presence of multiple cysts is also termed as congenital polycystic kidney.

Type-I cysts are formed due to dilation and hyperplasia of collecting tubules resulting in spongiform kidneys. In such neonates cystic bile ducts are also present.

Type-II polycystic kidney is formed due to absence of collecting tubules and developmental failure of nephron. The cysts are thick walled with dense connective tissue and may involve one or both kidneys.

Type-III cysts in kidneys occur due to multiple abnormalities during development. Cysts develop from tubules or Bowmen's capsule with part of glomeruli in cyst. This condition is bilateral and causes considerable enlargement of kidney due to clear fluid or blood mixed fluid containing cysts.

Functional Disturbances

Proteinuria

Presence of protein particularly albumin in urine. Protein is found as smooth, homogenous, pink staining precipitate also called as 'cast'. The presence of albumin in urine is indicative of damage in glomeruli. It is also characterized by oedema due to protein deficiency.

Hematuria

Presence of blood in urine giving bright red colour. It may occur due to damage in glomeruli, tubule or hemorrhage anywhere from glomeruli to urethra. The most important cause of hematuria is bracken fern toxicity (Fig. 7.1).

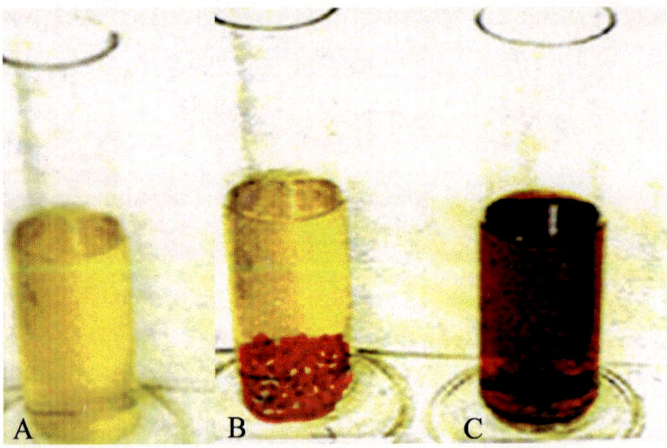

Fig. 7.1: Photograph showing (A) Normal (B) hematuria and (C) hemoglobinuria

Hemoglobinuria

When hemoglobin is present in urine without erythrocytes due to intravascular hemolysis. The urine becomes brownish red in colour. It must be differentiated from hematuria in which intact erythrocytes are present and settle down after some time leaving clear urine as supernatant. Hemoglobinuria is caused by various infections such as *Leptospira* sp., Babesia sp. or phosphorus deficiency in animals (Fig. 7.1).

Anuria

Absence of urine is known as anuria which may be due to:

- Absence of urinary secretion due to glomerulonephritis.

- Inelastic renal capsule unable to exert sufficient pressure required for glomerular filtration leading to nephrosis.
- Due to hydronephrosis or calculi urine already secreted puts back pressure to prevent further secretion.
- Low blood pressure.
- Dehydration.
- Necrosis of tubular epithelium.

Polyuria

Increased amount of urine leading to frequent urination caused due to diabetes insipidus, hormonal imbalance and polydipsia. In this condition, waste products are successfully eliminated.

Uremia

The presence of harmful waste products like uric acid, creatinine and urea in blood. Normally such waste products are removed by excretion through kidneys. But due to damage in kidneys or obstruction by inflammation, neoplasm, abscess and most importantly by presence of calculi, urine remains in the system and causes uremia. Uremia is characterized by headache, vomiting, hyperirritability, convulsion, ulcers in oral cavity and stomach, normochromic and normocytic anemia, hemosiderosis and thrombocytopenia.

Glycosuria

Presence of glucose in urine. This is also known as diabetes mellitus, a metabolic disorder. It may occur due to insulin deficiency. This condition is not common in animals. However, it may occur in dogs as a result of hypoglycemia. It may occur in sheep due to enterotoxaemia caused by *Clostridium welchii* type D.

Pyuria

Presence of pus in urine due to suppurative inflammation in urinary tract.

Ketonuria

Presence of ketone bodies in urine, which is common in diabetes mellitus, acetonemia, pregnancy toxaemia and in starvation.

Oliguria

In this condition, there is decreased amount of urine, which occurs due to glomerulonephritis, obstruction in urinary passage, dehydration, low blood pressure and tubular damage.

Nephrosis

Nephrosis is the degeneration and necrosis of tubular epithelium without producing inflammatory reaction. It mostly includes acute tubular necrosis as a result of ischemia or toxic injury to kidney. Nephrosis is characterized by necrosis and sloughing of tubular epithelial cells exhibited by uremia, oliguria, anuria (Figs. 7.2 to 7.4).

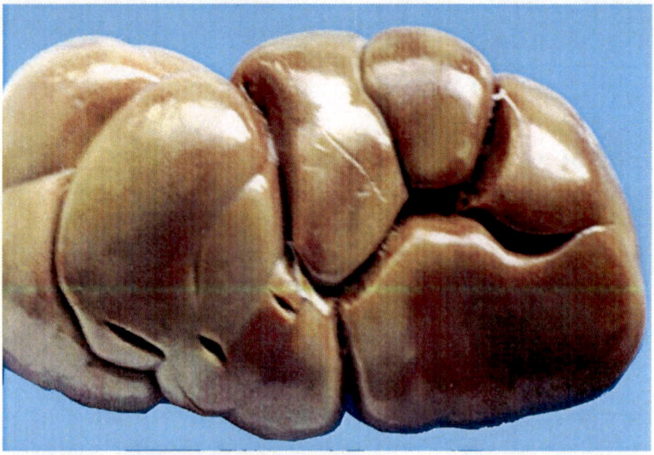

Fig. 7.2: Photograph showing nephrosis

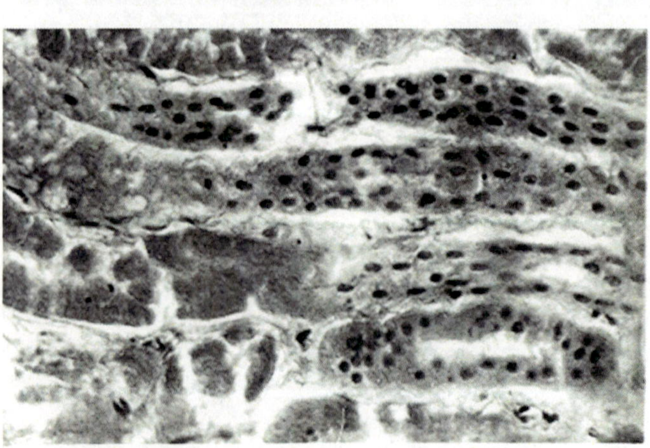

Fig. 7.3: Photomicrograph showing nephrosis

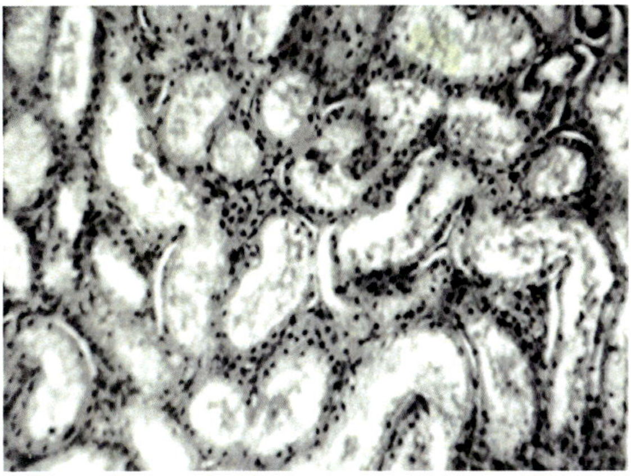

Fig. 7.4: Photomicrograph showing nephrosis

Etiology

- Hypotension.
- Heavy metals.
- Mycotoxins e.g. Ochratoxin.
- Antibiotics e.g. Gentamicin.

Macroscopic features

- Swelling of kidneys.
- Capsular surface smooth, pale and translucent.

Microscopic features

- Vacuolation in tubular epithelium.
- Coagulative necrosis.
- Sloughing of tubular epithelium.

Glomerulonephritis

Glomerulonephritis is the inflammation of glomeruli primarily characterized by pale and enlarged kidneys with potential hemorrhage, oedema of glomeruli, congestion and infiltration of inflammatory cells. Due to presence of mesangial proliferation, it is also called mesangio proliferative glomerulonephritis (MPGN) (Figs. 7.5 to 7.7).

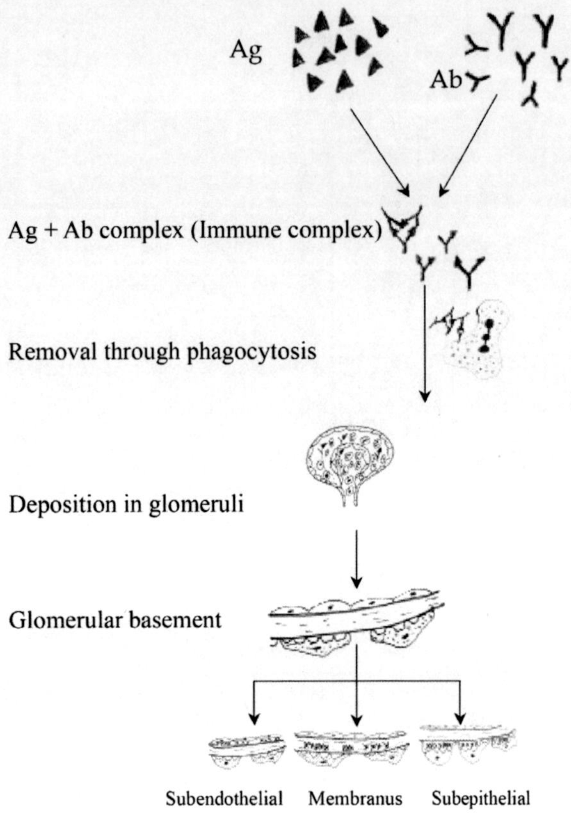

Fig. 7.5: Diagram of immune complex mediated glomerulone

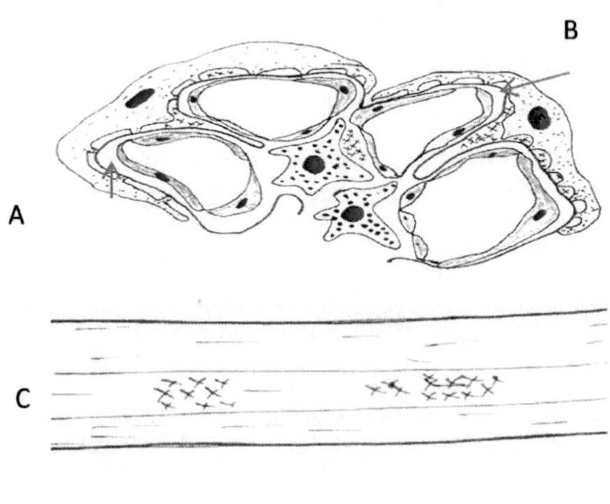

Fig. 7.6: Diagram showing different locations of deposits of immune complexes A. subendothelial B. Membranous and C. Sub epithelial deposits of immune complexes.

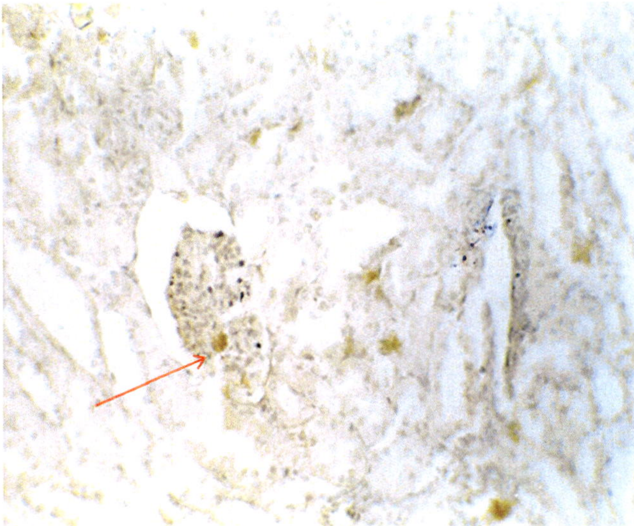

Fig. 7.7: Photomicrograph showing immune complexes in glomeruli (Immunoperoxidase staining)

Etiology

- Streptococci infection.
- Immune complexes.
- Environmental pollutants such as Organochlorine pesticides.

Macroscopic features

- Enlarged kidneys.
- Oedema, pale kidneys.
- Petechiae on kidneys.
- Proteinuria, uremia, hypercholesterolemia and increased creatinine level in blood.

Microscopic features

- Oedema of glomeruli leading to increase in size.
- Infiltration of neutrophils, macrophages.
- Compression of blood capillaries and absence of erythrocytes.
- Thrombosis and necrosis of glomerular capillaries.

Based on type of lesions, it can be divided into 5 subtypes.

1. Type-I MPGN

- Proliferation of mesangial cells.
- Deposition of immune complexes containing IgG, IgM, IgA and C_3.
- Immune complexes penetrate vascular endothelium but not the basement membrane and are deposited in subendothelial region.
- Proliferation and swelling of endothelial cells.
- Immune complexes induce production of transforming growth factor ($TGFB_1$) which increases production of fibrinolectin, collagen and proteoglycans leading to thickness of basement membrane; this is also known as "wire loop" lesions.

2. Type-II MPGN (Membranous)

- Deposition of immune complexes in basement membrane (lamina densa).
- Due to uncontrolled activation of complement.
- Proliferation of endothelium and mesangial cells.
- Demonstration of C_3 component, no immunoglobulin.

3. Type III MPGN (Acute Proliferative)

- Subepithelial deposits of immune complexes and disruption of basement membrane.
- Swelling of epithelium and its proliferation forming "Epithelial cresent".
- Demonstration of IgG in subepithelial region.
- Congestion and oedema of glomeruli.
- Infiltration of neutrophils, macrophages and lymphocytes.

4. Chronic glomerulonephritis

- Proliferation of epithelial and endothelial cells.
- Reduplication, thickening and disorganization of glomerular basement membrane.
- Lumen of capillaries occluded.
- Entire glomerulus is replaced by Hyaline connective tissue.

5. Focal embolic glomerulonephritis

- Focal zone of necrosis in glomeruli.
- Infiltration of neutrophils.
- Proliferation of epithelial cells and formation of crescent.

Interstitial Nephritis

Interstitial nephritis is the inflammation of kidney characterized by degeneration and necrosis of tubular epithelium, oedema and infiltration of inflammatory cells in interstitium (Figs. 7.8 & 7.9).

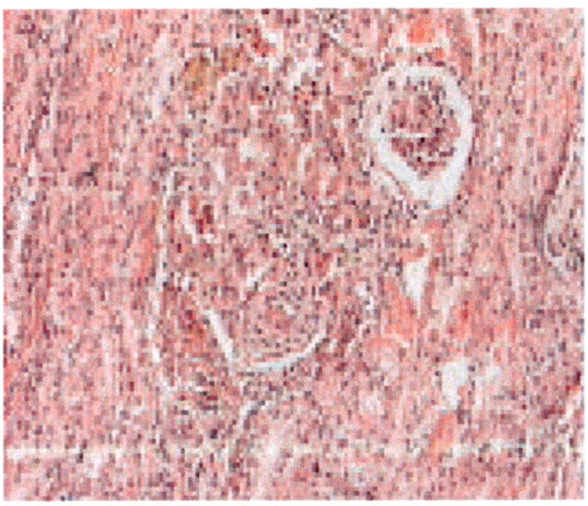

Fig. 7.8: Photomicrograph showing interstitial nephritis.

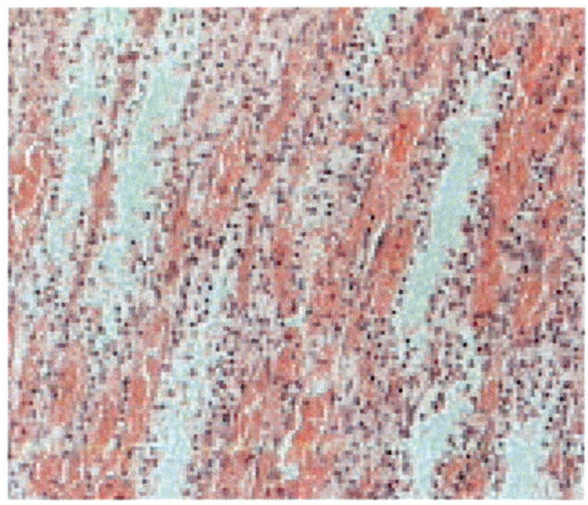

Fig. 7.8: Photomicrograph showing interstitial nephritis

Etiology

- Ochratoxins and atrinin.
- Leptospira.
- Toxins/ poisons e.g. pesticides.
- Herpes virus.
- Endogenous toxaemia e.g. ketosis.
- Immune complexes.

Macroscopic features

- Enlargement of kidneys.
- Necrosis, congestion and hemorrhage.

Microscopic features

- Oedema, congestion, hemorrhage.
- Necrosis and degeneration of tubular epithelium.
- Infiltration of inflammatory cells like neutrophils, macrophages and lymphocytes in interstitium.
- Loss of tubules, foci of mononuclear cells, fibrosis in chronic cases.
- Immune complexes are deposited in granular form causing degeneration of epithelial cells of tubules and mononuclear cell infiltration.

Pyelonephritis

Pyelonephritis is the inflammation of renal pelvis and parenchyma i.e. tubules characterized by congestion, suppurative inflammation and fibrosis.

Etiology

- Corynebacterium renale.
- Staphylococcus aureus.
- *E. coli.*
- Actinomyces pyogenes.
- Pseudomonas aeruginosa.

Macroscopic features

- Congestion, hemorrhage and abscess formation in renal cortex, pelvis and ureters.
- Pyuria – pus mixed urine in bladder.
- Enlargement of kidneys.

Microscopic features

- Congestion, hemorrhage. Suppurative inflammation of pelvis and kidney parenchyma (Fig. 7.10).
- Necrosis of collecting ducts.
- Purulent exudate in pelvis.
- Infiltration of neutrophils, lymphocytes and plasma cells in interstitium.

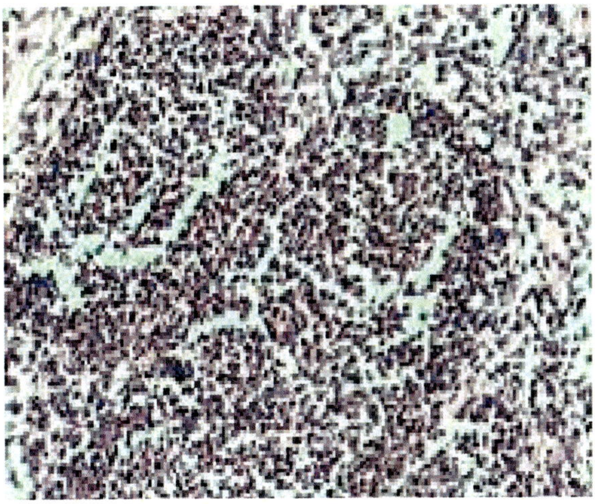

Fig. 7.10: Photomicrograph showing suppurative nephritis

Table 7.1: Differential features of various types of Nephritis

	Glomerulonephritis	**Interstitial**	**Pyelonephritis**
Macroscopic features	1. Enlarged kidneys 2. Oedema, pale kidneys 3. Petechiae on kidneys 4. Proteinuria, uremia, hypercholesterolemia and increased creatinine level in blood.	1. Enlargement of kidneys 2. Necrosis, congestion and Hemorrhage	1. Congestion, hemorrhage and abscess formation in renal cortex, pelvis and ureters. 2. Pyuria- Pus mixed urine in bladder. 3. Enlargement of kidneys
Microscopic features	1. Oedema of glomeruli leading to increase in size. 2. Infiltration of neutrophils, macrophages. 3. Compression of blood capillaries and absence of erythrocytes. 4. Thrombosis and necrosis of glomerular capillaries.	1. Oedema, congestion, Haemorrhage 2. Necrosis and degeneration of tubular epithelium 3. Infiltration of inflammatory cells like neutrophils, macrophages and lymphocytes in interstitium.	1. Congestion, haemorrhage 2. Suppurative inflammation of pelvis and kidney parenchyma. 3. Necrosis of collecting ducts. 4. Purulent exudate in pelvis.

	Glomerulonephritis	Interstitial	Pyelonephritis
		4. Loss of tubules, foci of mononuclear cells, fibrosis in chronic cases 5. Immune complexes are deposited in granular form causing degeneration of epithelial cells of tubules and mononuclear cell infiltration.	5. Infiltration of neutrophils, lymphocytes and plasma cells in interstitium.

Nephrosclerosis

Nephrosclerosis is chronic fibrosis of kidney characterized by loss of glomeruli and tubules and extensive fibrosis (Fig. 7.11).

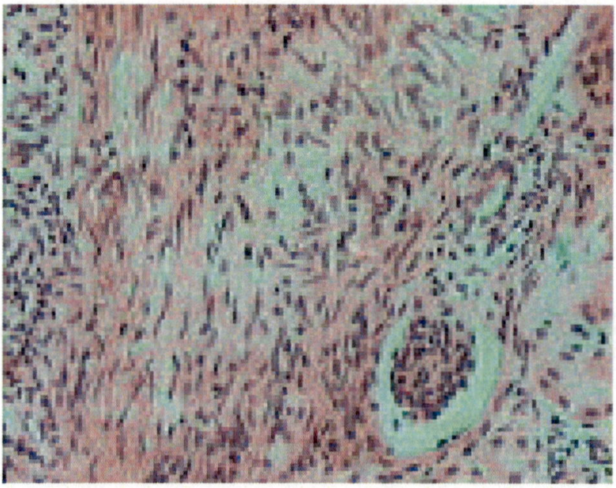

Fig. 7.11: Photomicrograph of kidney showing nephrosclerosis

Etiology

- Glomerulonephritis.
- Interstitial nephritis.
- Arterioloscleresis.

Macroscopic features

- Hard, atrophied kidneys.
- Fibrous nodules on kidneys.
- Thickening of capsule.
- Small white firm kidneys.

Microscopic features

- Ischemia, tubular atrophy.
- Loss of glomeruli and tubules.
- Extensive fibrosis.
- Deposition of hyaline mass.
- Infiltration of mononuclear cells.

Urolithiasis

Urolithiasis is the formation of stony precipitates anywhere in the urinary passage including kidneys, ureter, urinary bladder or urethra.

Etiology

- Bacterial infections.
- Metabolic defects.
- Vitamin A deficiency.
- Hyperparathyroidism.
- Mineral imbalance.

Macroscopic features

- Nephrosis, hydronephrosis.
- Distension of ureters.
- Distension of ureters and urinary bladder.
- Hard enlarged kidneys.

Presence of calculi/ stone in kidney, ureter, bladder or urethra (Figs. 7.12 & 7.14).

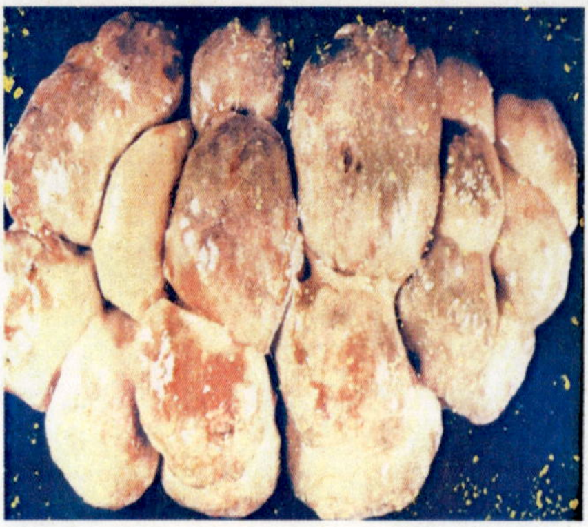

Fig.7.12: Photograph of kidney showing nephrolithiasis

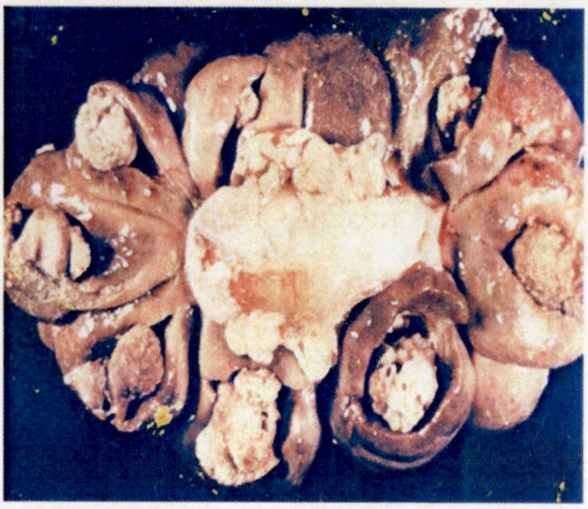

Fig. 7.13: Photograph of kidney showing nephrolithiasis

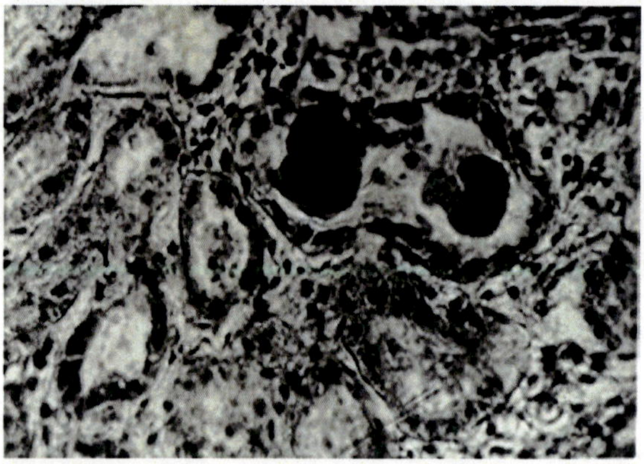

Fig. 7.14: Photomicrograph of kidney showing nephrolithiasis

There are various types of calculi, which differ in size, shape and composition. Some of them are as under:

Oxalate calculi are hard, light yellow, covered with sharp spines, found in urinary bladder and formed by calcium oxalate. They cause damage in urinary bladder leading to hemorrhage.

Uric acid calculi are composed of ammonium and sodium urates and uric acids, are yellow to brown in colour, formed in acidic urine, are spherical and irregular in shape and are not radio opaque.

Phosphate calculi are white or grey in colour, chalky in consistency, soft, friable and can be crushed with mild pressure. They are mostly multiple in the form of sand-like granules. They are composed of magnesium ammonium phosphate and occur as a result of bacterial infection.

Xanthine calculi are brownish red, concentrically laminated, fragile and irregular in shape. They rarely occur in animals.

Cystine calculi are small, soft with shiny and greasy in appearance, yellow in colour which becomes darker on exposure to air. Insoluble amino acid cystine precipitates in bladder to form calculi. Such calculi may cause obstruction of urethra with cystinuria.

Microscopic features

- Presence of crystals/stone in lumen of tubules.
- Degeneration and necrosis of tubular epithelium.
- Hemorrhage.
- Proliferation of fibrous tissue.

Pathology of Ureter

Ureteritis

Ureteritis is the inflammation of ureter characterized by enlargement, thickening of wall due to accumulation of urates, or calculi, pyonephrosis and pyelonephritis (Fig. 7.15).

- Etiology
- Tuberculosis.
- Calculi.
- Hydronephrosis.
- Pyelonephritis.
- Pyonephrosis.

Macroscopic features

- Deposits of whitish/yellowish urates in ureter in poultry.
- Obstructions of ureter due to calculi leads to its enlargement and formation of diverticulum.

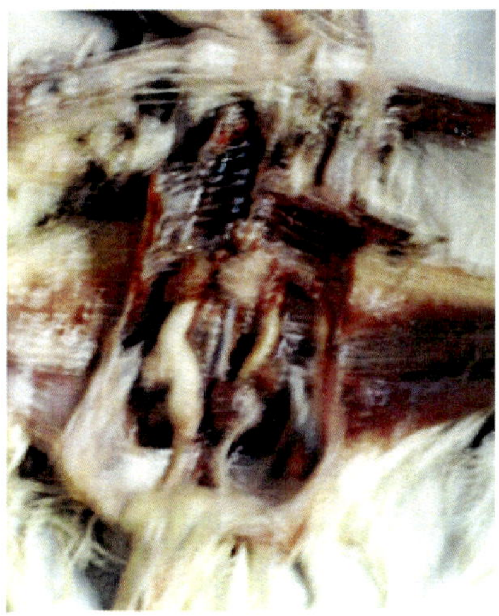

Fig. 7.15: Photograph showing ureteritis due to deposition of salts

Microscopic features

- Thickening of the wall due to congestion and infiltration of inflammatory cells.
- Extensive fibrosis with infiltration of mononuclear cells in chronic cases.

Pathology of Urinary Bladder

Cystitis

Cystitis is the inflammation of urinary bladder characterized by congestion and fibrinous, purulent or hemorrhagic exudate (Fig. 7.16).

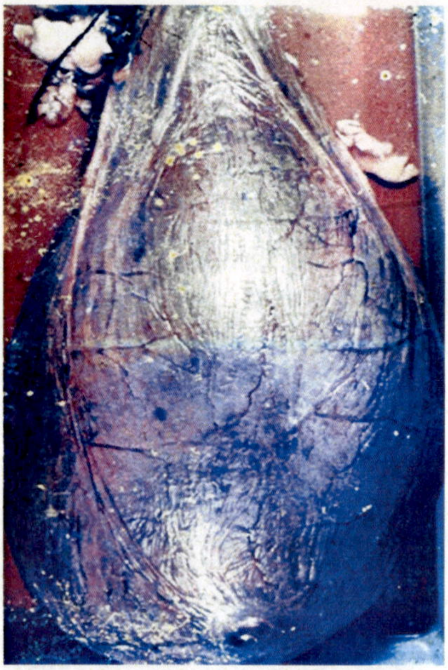

Fig. 7.16: Photograph showing cystitis

Etiology

- Urinary calculi.
- Tuberculosis.
- Blockage in urethra.
- Bracken fern poisoning.

Macroscopic features

- Congestion, hemorrhage.
- Enlargement of urinary bladder.
- Thickening of the wall.
- Presence of small nodules on wall.

Microscopic features

- Congestion, hemorrhage.
- Thickening of wall due to infiltration of neutrophils and macrophages.
- Granuloma in tuberculosis.
- Fibrosis
- Presence of neoplasm.

Pathology of Urethra

Urethritis

Inflammation of urethra is known as urethritis, which occurs as a result of catheter injury or calculi. It is characterized by congestion, obstruction, hydronephrosis and strictures (Fig. 7.17).

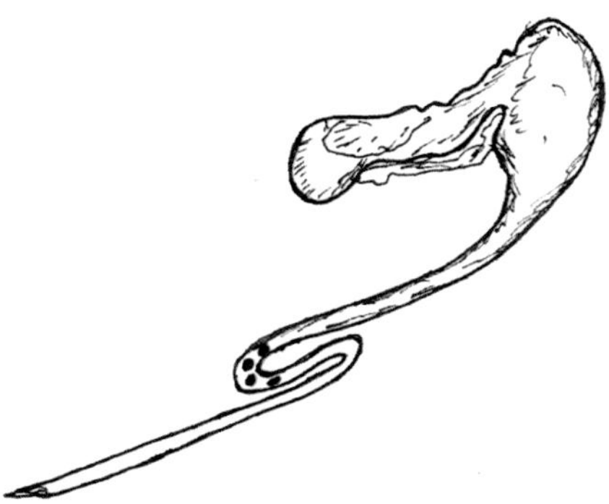

Fig. 7.17: Diagram showing retention of calculi in urethra of bovines.

Etiology

- Calculi.
- Catheter injury.
- Trichomonas foetus infection.
- Picorna virus infection.

Macroscopic features

- Transient inflammation, congestion and hemorrhage.
- Strictures (male), diverticulum (female).
- Obstruction due to calculi, presence of calculi.

Microscopic features

Thickening due to inflammatory exudate.

8

Pathology of Genital System

Female Genital System

Developmental Anomalies

Agenesis

Absence of ovary, uterus, oviduct and cervix in females. It may be unilateral or bilateral.

Hypoplasia

Complete or partial lack of germ cells in ovaries. Hypoplasia of uterus is related with agenesis of gonads. Ovaries of freemartin are also hypoplastic. Hermaphrodite animal has ovary and testicular tissue both in the gonads.

Hermaphroditism

In hermaphrodites, there is presence of organs of both sexes in same individual animal. Both ovarian and testicular tissue occur in one animal leads to sterility in animal (true hermaphrodite) while in pseudohermaphrodite the gonadal tissue of only one sex is present but there is some degree of development of opposite sex organs.

Uterus unicornis

Uterus unicornis is presence of only one horn of uterus instead of two, seen in animals with white heifer disease.

White heifer disease

White heifer disease occurs due to a single sex linked gene defect responsible for white coat colour. In such animals, there are normal ovaries, oviduct but uterus is incomplete and may lack communication with cervix. There is hypoplasia of cervix and vagina.

Uterus didelphys

Uterus didelphys is the occurrence of two cervix with two uterine bodies and single or double vagina. It occurs due to failure of mullerian ducts to fuse at their distal end. Sometimes failure of fusion may affect only cervix and there are two cervix which termed as Cervix bifida.

Cystic Ovaries

Cystic ovaries are defined as an ovary, which contains one or more clear cysts ranging from one to several centimeters in size (Fig. 8.1).

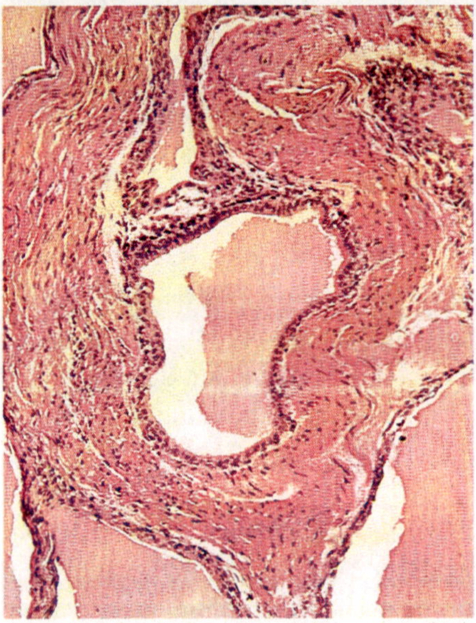

Fig. 8.1: Photomicrograph showing cystic ovary

Etiology

- Hormonal imbalance

Macroscopic features

- Presence of cysts in ovaries.
- Hormonal imbalance of animal leads to sterility, continuous estrus, nymphomania due to follicular cyst.
- Lutein cysts may cause pyometra leading to pseudopregnancy.

Microscopic features

- Follicular cyst.
- Ova absent several layers of granulosa or a single layer of epithelium.
- Many follicular cysts are present.
- Lutein cyst covered by fat containing granulosa cells.

Oophoritis

Oophoritis is the inflammation of ovary caused by trauma, infection and characterized by granulomatous or lymphocytic inflammation of ovary (Figs. 8.2 to 8.4).

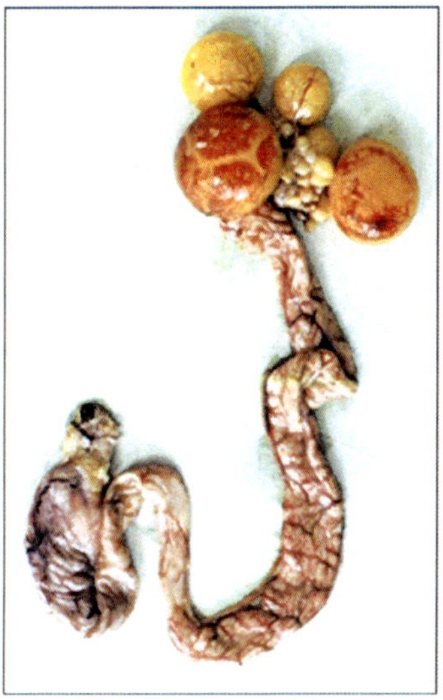

Fig. 8.2: Photograph showing oophoritis and salpingtis

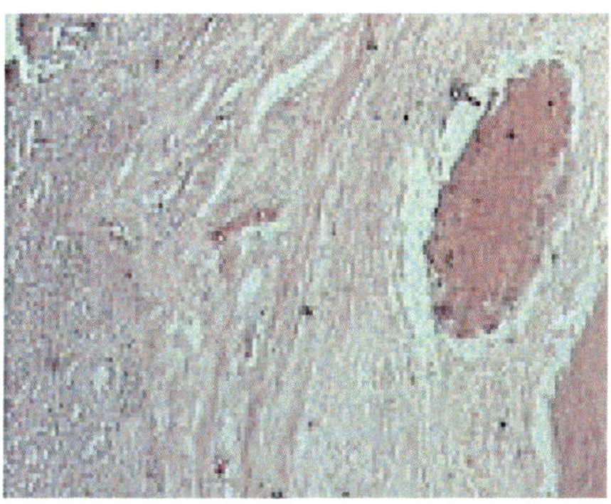

Fig. 8.3: Photomicrograph showing oophoritis

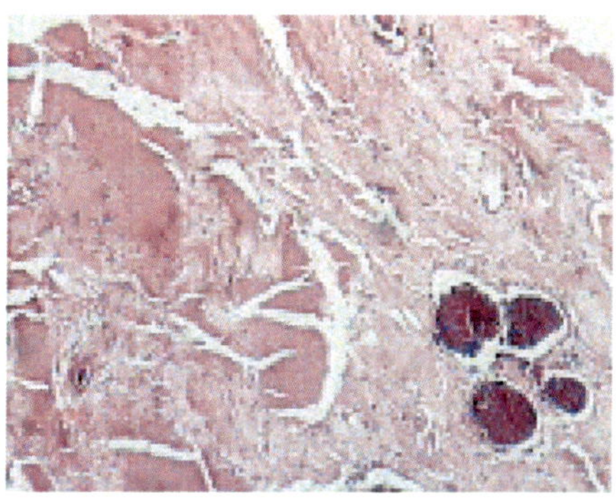

Fig. 8.4: Photomicrograph showing oophoritis

Etiology

- *Mycobacterium tuberculosis*.
- Herpes virus.

Macroscopic features

- Hard, nodular lesions in ovary, encapsulated with fibrous tissue.

Microscopic features

- Granuloma of tuberculosis through hematogenous infection.
- Infiltration of lymphocytes leading to lymphofollicular reaction in follicles.
- Atrophy or absence of ova.

Salpingitis

Salpingitis is the inflammation of oviduct or fallopian tube characterized by congestion, catarrhal or purulent exudate leading to distended lumen (Fig. 8.2).

Etiology

- Mycoplasma.
- Streptococci.
- Tuberculosis (*Mycobacterium tuberculosis*).
- Trichomoniasis (*Trichomonas foetus*).

Macroscopic features

- Congestion, abscess formation
- Distension of oviduct lumen due to accumulation of serous exudate which is known as Hydrosalpinx.
- Accumulation of pus in oviduct is termed as Pyosalpinx.
- Fibrosis, hardness.
- Occlusion of lumen due to inflammatory exudate resulting in sterility.
- Inflammatory exudate is toxic to ova as well as sperms leading to sterility.

Microscopic features

- Congestion.
- Suppurative inflammation.
- Infiltration of neutrophils, macrophages and lymphocytes.
- Proliferation of fibrous tissue.
- Debris of desquamated cells.

Metritis

Metritis is the inflammation of uterus characterized by suppurative exudate, hemorrhage and necrosis of uterus (Fig. 8.5).

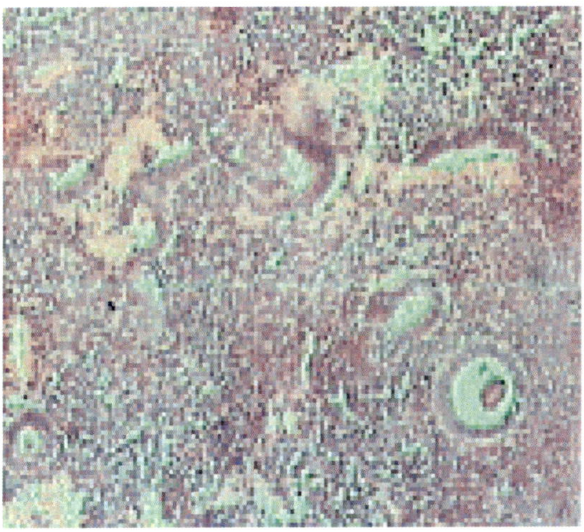

Fig. 8.5: Photomicrograph showing metritis

Etiology

- *Actinomyces pyogenes.*
- *E. coli.*
- Staphylococci.
- Streptococci.
- *Trichomonas foetus.*
- *Campylobacter foetus.*

Macroscopic features

- Congestion, catarrhal or purulent exudate.
- Hemorrhage.
- Enlargement, oedema.
- Oozing out of pus from uterus on pressure.

Microscopic features

- Seropurulent exudate in uterine wall.
- Oedema.
- Infiltration of macrophages and lymphocytes.
- Desquamation of lining epithelium.

Pyometra

Pyometra is an acute or chronic suppurative inflammation of uterus resulting in accumulation of pus in the uterus.

Etiology

- Occurs under the influence of progesterone.
- *E. coli.*
- *Actinomyces pyogenes.*
- *Proteus* spp.
- *Staphylococcus aureus.*
- *Trichomonas foetus.*

Macroscopic features

- Discharge of thin cream like pus from vulva soiling the tail and perineal region.
- Pus discharge is more on sitting position of animal.
- Enlargement of abdomen due to distension of uterus.
- Uterus looking like a pregnant uterus as a result of accumulation of pus. This condition is also known as Pseudocyesis or pseudopregnancy.
- Retention of lutein cyst.

Microscopic features

- Congestion, infiltration of neutrophils, lymphocytes and plasma cells.
- Necrosis of mucosal epithelium of uterus.
- Proliferation of endometrial epithelium.
- Oedema, glandular hyperplasia.

Endometritis

Endometritis is the inflammation of endometrium, the mucosa of uterus. It may be catarrhal or purulent and may occur after metritis.

Etiology

- Trichomonas foetus.
- Campylobacter foetus.
- Staphylococci.
- Streptococci.
- Organism enters in uterus as a result of coitus, artificial insemination or as iatrogenic infection.
- Strong chemicals/medicines administered in uterus.

Macroscopic features

- Catarrhal discharge from uterus containing desquamated cells.
- Sterility due to toxic environment of uterus to sperms.
- Congestion.

Microscopic features

- Congestion.
- Moderate infiltration of lymphocytes, plasma cells and neutrophils in mucosa.

Cervicitis

Cervicitis is the inflammation of cervix as a result of either descending infection from uterus or ascending infection from vagina and characterized by catarrhal inflammation.

Etiology

- Etiological agents are similar as in endometritis.

Macroscopic features

- Congestion.
- Enlargement of cervix.

Microscopic features

- Catarrhal inflammation of cervical mucosa.
- Hyperplasia of mucous glands with tall mucin containing epithelial cells.
- Presence of mucin in lumen.

Vaginitis

Vaginitis is the inflammation of vagina characterized by congestion, granularity as a result of elevations in mucosa. This is also known as infectious pustular vulvovaginitis in cattle caused by herpes virus.

Etiology

- Mycoplasma bovigenitalium.
- Bovine herpes virus-1 (BHV-1).
- Picorna virus.
- *Trichomonas foetus*.

Macroscopic features

- Granular elevation in vaginal mucosa.
- Congestion (Fig. 8.6).

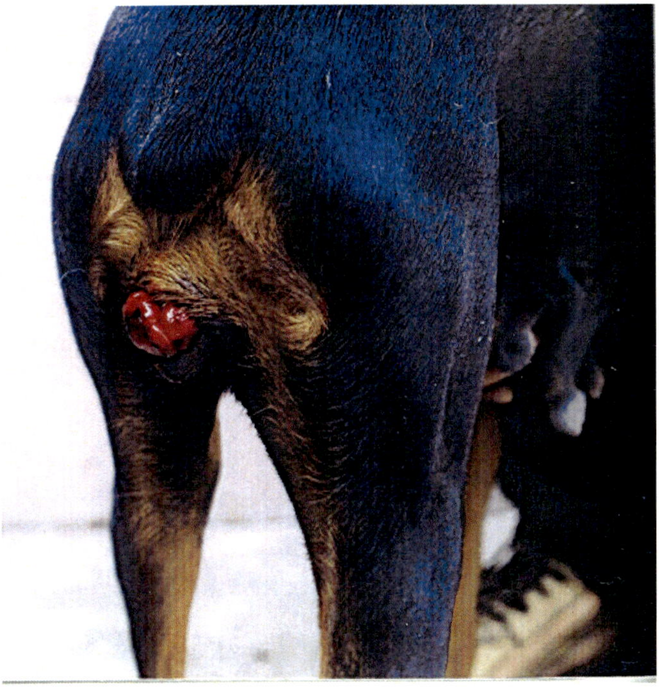

Fig. 8.6: Photograph showing prolapse of vagina

- Prolapse due to inflammation (Fig. 8.7).

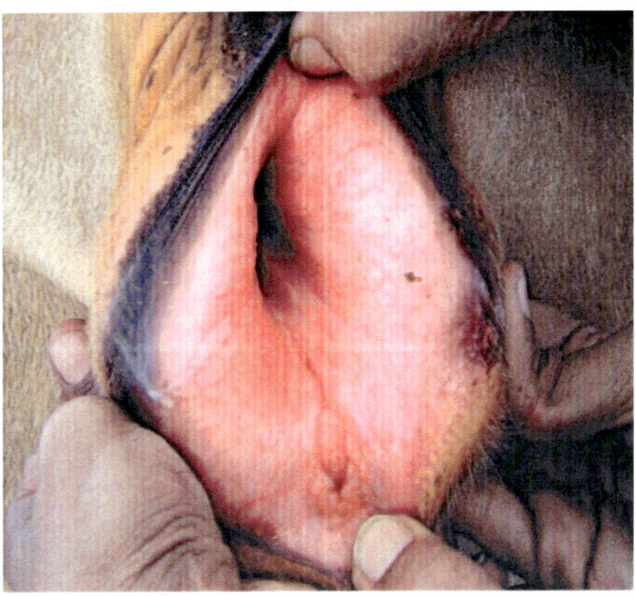

Fig. 8.7: Vaginitis due to bovine herpes virus-1

Microscopic features

- Accumulation of lymphocytes in sub-epithelial region.
- Congestion.

Abortion

Abortion is expulsion of dead embryo or foetus before attaining normal gestation. There are two other terms related to abortion i.e. stillbirth and premature birth. Stillbirth is defined as expulsion of dead foetus on its full maturity while premature birth is birth of a live foetus before attaining full gestation period.

Etiology

- Brucellosis (*Brucella abortus, B. meletensis, B. ovis*).
- Campylobacter foetus.
- *Salmonella abortus-equi* – mares.
- Equine herpes virus – mares.
- Bovine herpes virus-1 – cattle.
- *Chlamydia psittasci.*
- *Trichomonas foetus.*
- Listeria monocytogenes (Listeria ivanovii).
- *Leptospria* spp.
- *Mycobacterium tuberculosis.*
- *Toxoplasma gondii.*
- Mycoplasma mycoides.
- Fungi – *Aspergillus* spp., *Coccidioides* spp. *Absidia* spp.
- Toxins / poisons.

Macroscopic features

- Expulsion of dead foetus in early stage (3-4 month) of gestation (Trichomoniasis).
- Abortion in middle of gestation (Campylobacteriosis).
- Late abortions (7-9 months) occur due to Brucellosis, BHV-1 infection (Fig. 8.8).

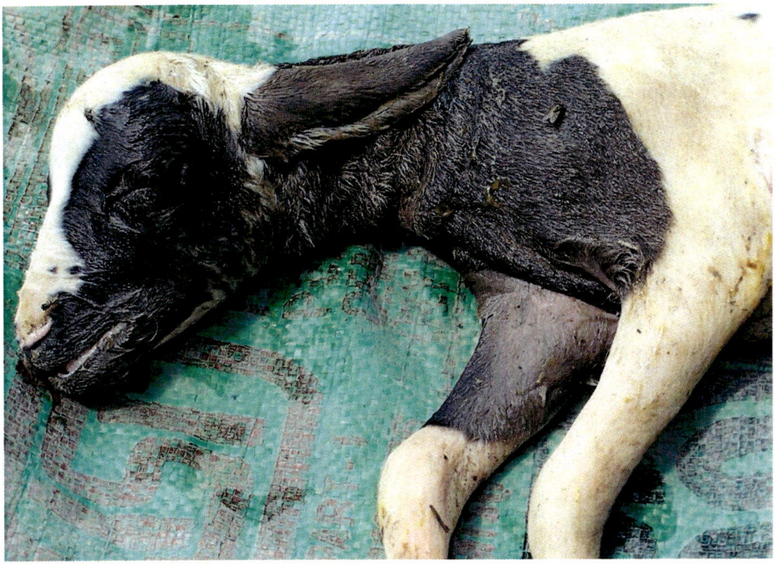

Fig. 8.8: Aborted foetus due to brucellosis

- Liver of foetus has necrotic foci, congestion.
- Stomach contents used for confirmation of etiology.
- In some cases of abortion, there is retention of placenta (e.g. Brucellosis).
- Placenta becomes oedematous and necrotic (Placentitis).
- If the foetus dies and is not expelled outside the body due to non-opening of cervix, the dead foetus remains in uterus under sterile conditions. Such foetus undergoes autolysis and is liquified. Liquid material is absorbed in uterus through lymph or blood but bones/skin etc. remain in uterine horn sometimes causing irritation or damage to endometrium. Such foetus becomes shrunken with wrinkled skin and dried as mummy and is known as "Mummified foetus".

Microscopic features

- Necrotic hepatitis with lymphofollicular reaction in foetus (Brucellosis, BHV-1 infection).
- Granulomatous lesions (tuberculosis, fungal infection), lymphofollicular reaction (mycoplasma, chlamydia).
- Demonstration/isolation of causative organisms in foetal stomach contents.

- Liver of foetus icteric (leptospirosis).
- Endometritis in dam.
- Bronchopneumonia in foetus e.g. brucellosis.

Retained Placenta/Placentitis

Retention of placenta occurs after abortion or parturition as a result of inflammation characterized by swelling, oedema or fibrosis which prevent the separation of chorion from endometrium (Figs. 8.9 & 8.10).

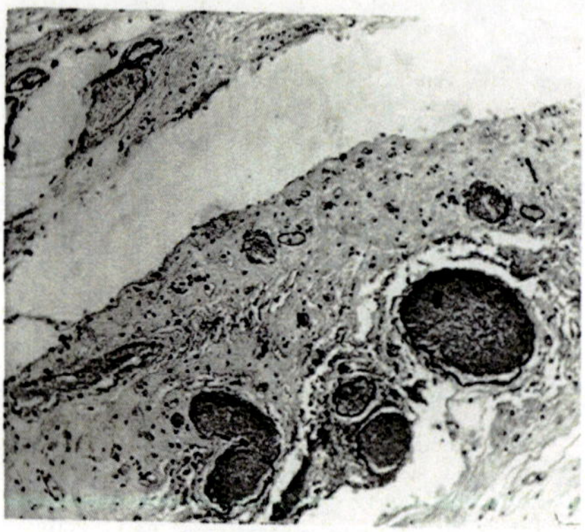

Fig. 8.9: Photomicrograph showing oedema and congestion in placenta (Placentitis) due to brucellosis

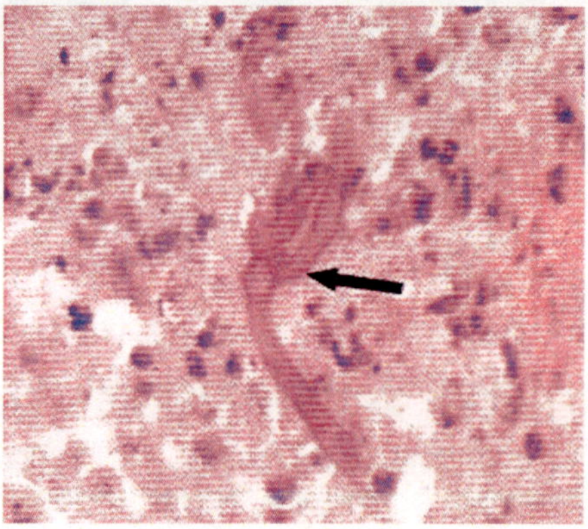

Fig. 8.10: Photomicrograph showing fungal placentitis

Etiology

- Lack of progesterone.
- Infection e.g. Brucellosis, Trichomoniasis.

Macroscopic features

- Retained placenta undergoes autolysis, putrefaction.
- Toxaemia in dam.
- Endometritis, pyometra.

Microscopic features

- Placenta is oedematous and congested.
- Infiltration of neutrophils, mononuclear cells.

- Proliferation of fibroblasts.

Mastitis

Mastitis is the inflammation of mammary gland characterized by oedema hemorrhage and fibrosis of udder. Mastitis is always infectious and is a disease of lactating glands. There is no hematogenous infection and infections enter through teat canal to cause mastitis (Figs. 8.11 to 8.15).

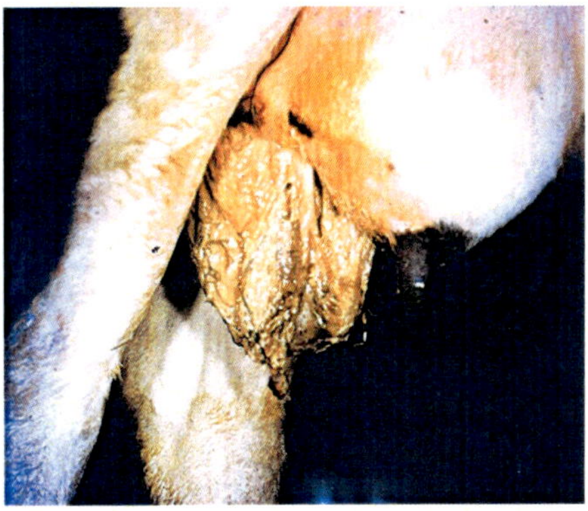

Fig. 8.11: Photograph showing mastitis due to fusarium toxicosis

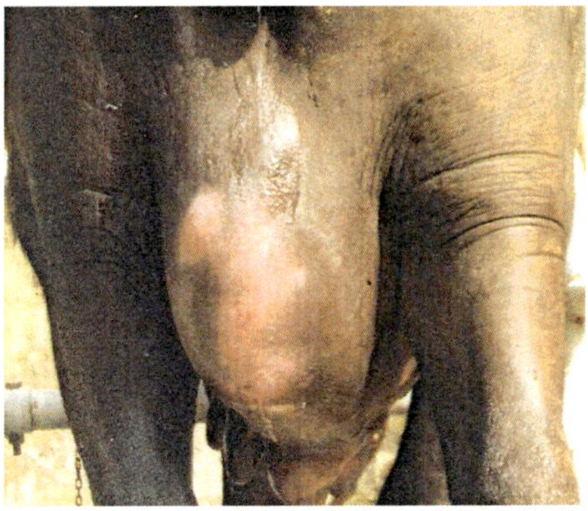

Fig. 8.12: Photograph of a buffalo suffering from Mastitis caused by pyogenic bacteria

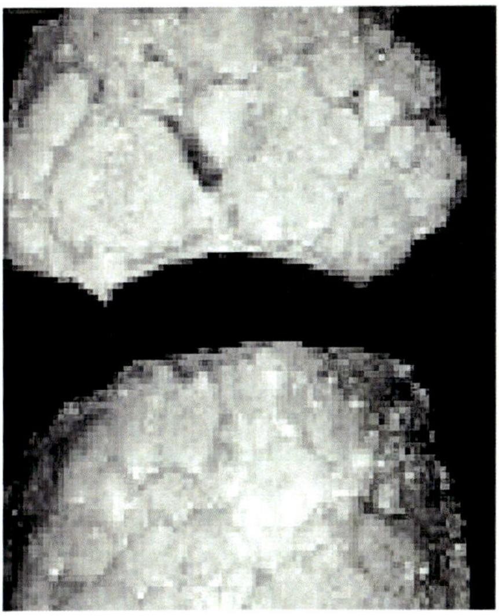

Fig. 8.13: Photograph showing chronic granulomatous mastitis

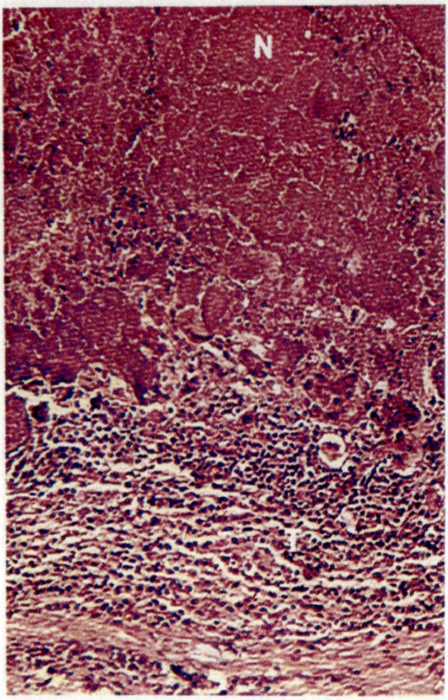

Fig. 8.14: Photomicrograph showing chronic granulomatous mastitis

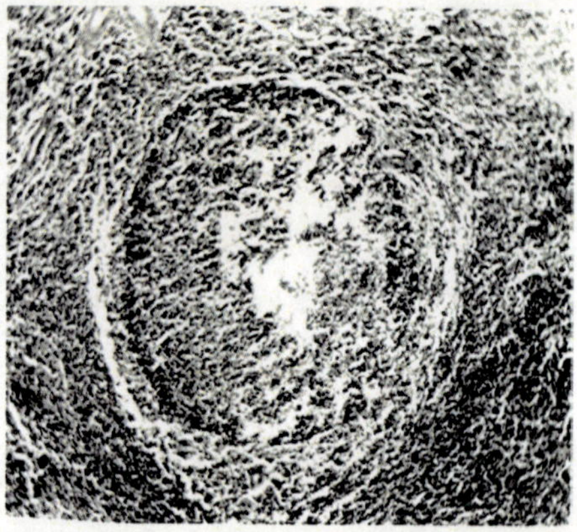

Fig. 8.15: Photomicrograph showing chronic granulomatous mastitis

Etiology

- Bacteria e.g. *Streptococcus agalactiae, Streptococcus dysgalactiae, Staphylococcus aureus, Actinomyces pyogenes, Pseudomonas aeruginosa, Brucella abortus, Mycobacterium tuberculosis, E. coli, Pasteurella multocida* and many more.
- Virus e.g. FMD virus, pox virus, BHV-1.
- Mycoplasma e.g. *Mycoplasma mycoides*.
- Fungi e.g. *Candida ablicans, Trichosporon* spp. *Nocardia asteroids, Cryptococcus neoformans.*

Macroscopic features

- Oedema of udder.
- Flakes (coagulated milk proteins) in milk.
- Blood mixed milk.

- Watery dirty grey or dark colour milk in animals. In dry period it is caused by *Actinomyces pyogenes* and is known as "summer mastitis".
- Terminal atrophy or shrunken quarter.
- Gangrene formation.

Microscopic features

- Congestion, hemorrhage.
- Infiltration of neutrophils, macrophages, lymphocytes.
- Necrosis of alveolar epithelium, hyperplasia of epithelial lining.
- Proliferation of fibrous tissue.
- Increase in WBC count in milk (more than 100/ml milk).

Male Genital System

Developmental Anomalies

Testicular hypoplasia

Testicular hypoplasia occurs in animals with chromosomal abnormality such as XXY chromosomes or Klinefelter's syndrome. Hypoplasia is also seen in hermaphrodites and in animals with cryptorchidism.

Spermatocele

There is failure of development of mesonephric tubules and it does not connect with vas deferens resulting in blind tubules filled with spermatozoa. Rupture of tubules may lead to spermatic granuloma.

Cryptorchidism

The testicles fail to descend in scrotum through inguinal canal after birth and remains in abdominal cavity. This permanent retention of testicles in abdominal cavity causes their hypoplasia leading to lack of spermatogenesis. Such testes are more prone to development of neoplastic growth.

Phimosis

Phimosis is the failure of extension of penis from its sheath.

Paraphimosis

Paraphimosis is the failure of withdrawal of extended penis.

Hypospadias

In hypospadias, there is urethral opening in ventral side of the penis.

Epispadias

There is urethral opening on the dorsal side of the penis.

Phallocampsis

Phallocampsis is the deviation of penis, which may be spiral (Cork screw penis) or ventral deviation (rainbow penis).

Orchitis

Orchitis is the inflammation of testes characterized by oedema, necrosis and infiltration of neutrophils, macrophages, lymphocytes and proliferation of fibrous tissue leading to atrophy in chronic cases (Figs. 8.16 to 8.20).

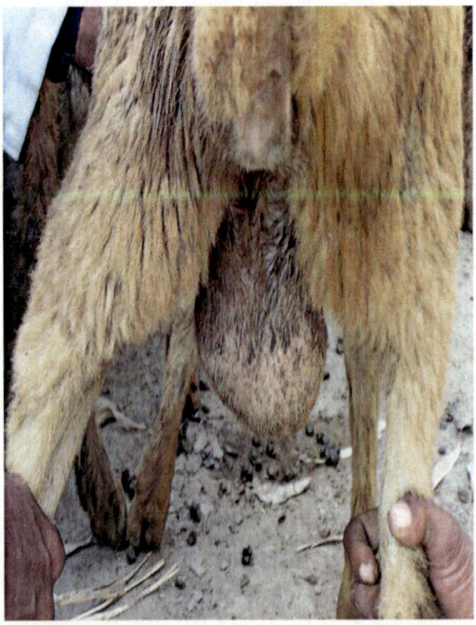

Fig. 8.16: Orchitis in ram due to brucellosis

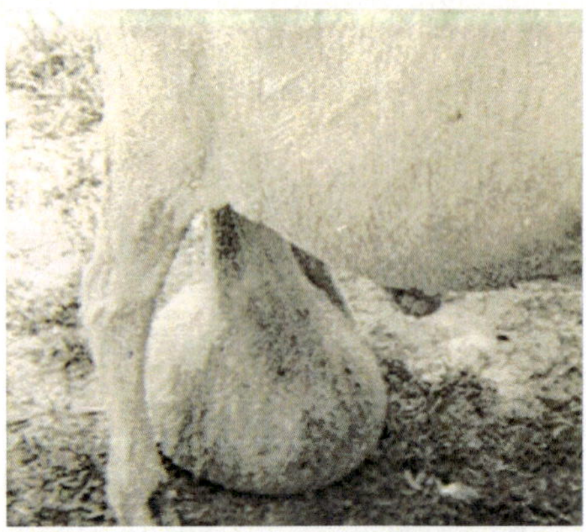

Fig. 8.17: Photograph showing orchitis in a ram

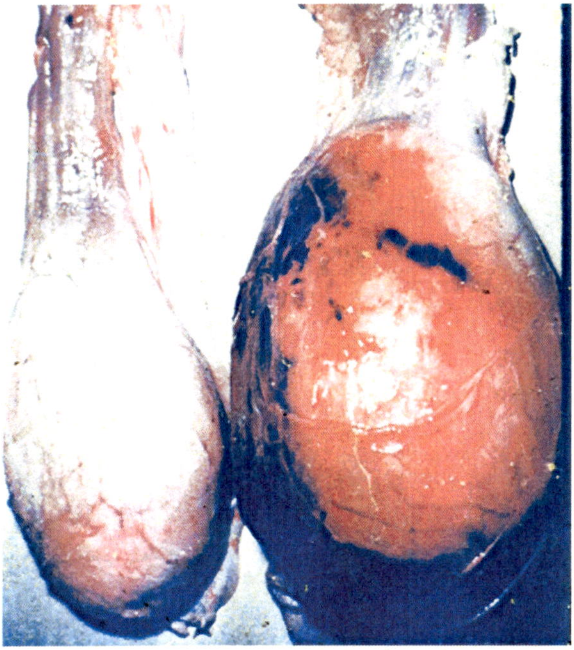

Fig. 8.18: Photograph of testicles showing (A) normal (b) Acute orchitis.

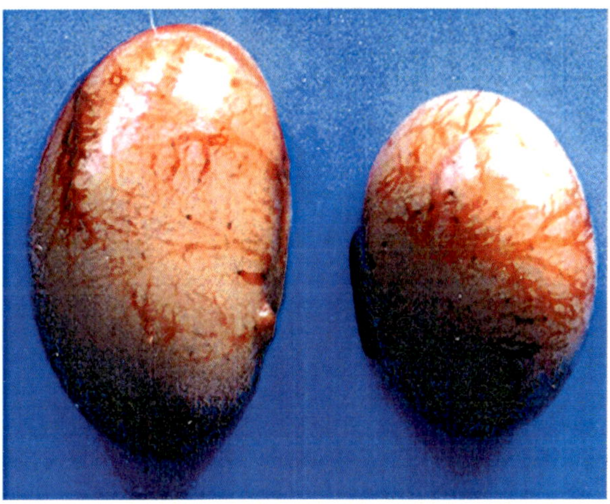

Fig. 8.19: Photograph of testicles of poultry showing orchitis due to salmonellosis

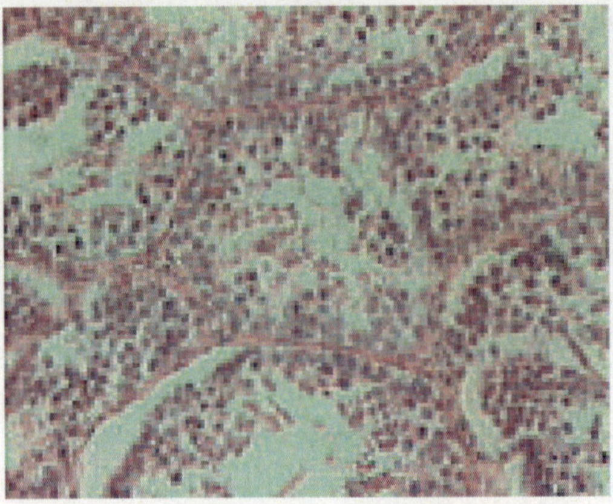

Fig. 8.20: Photomicrograph showing orchitis

Etiology

- *Brucella* spp.
- *Campylobactor* spp.
- *Salmonella* spp.
- *Trichomonas* spp.
- *Corynebacterium pseudotuberculosis.*
- *Actinomycess pyogenes.*
- *Pseudomanas aeruginosa.*
- *Actinomyces bovis.*

Macroscopic feature

- Enlargement of testes, oedema.
- Accumulation of serus fluid in scrotal sac/tunica vaginalis is called as hydrocele.
- Enlargement of scrotum.
- Congestion.
- Atrophy and hardening in chronic cases.

Microscopic features

- Congestion.

- Infiltration of neutrophils and mononuclear cells.
- Necrosis of germinal cells.
- Proliferation of fibrous tissue and infiltration of mononuclear cells.
- Granulomatous lesions in case of actinomycosis and tuberculosis.
- Aspermatogenesis.

Epididymitis

Epididymitis is the inflammation of epididymis characterized by catarrhal or suppurative exudate with necrosis of lining epithelium.

Etiology

- *Brucella ovis* in sheep.
- Other organisms that cause orchitis which is preceded by epididymitis.

Macroscopic features

- Enlargement of epididymis.
- Oedema of scrotum.
- Accumulation of mucus and/or purulent exudate in epididymis.
- Accumulation of serus exudate in scrotum.

Microscopic features

- Necrosis of lining epithelium of epididymis.
- Infiltration of neutrophils, macrophages and lymphocytes.
- Oedema.
- Formation of granuloma in chronic cases.

Funiculitis

Funiculitis is inflammation of scirrhous cord characterized by enlargement of scrotum due to chronic abscess.

Etiology/Occurrence

- Botryomycosis.
- Actinomycosis.

- Castration.
- Unsanitary conditions.

Macroscopic features

- Enlargement of scrotum.
- Hard swelling/ chronic abscess.

Microscopic features

- Chronic hyperplastic/proliferative changes.
- Fibroplasia.
- Infiltration of macrophages, lymphocytes, neutrophils around sulfur granules forming rosette.

Seminal Vesiculitis

Seminal vesiculitis is the inflammation of seminal vesicle characterized by metaplasia of the columnar epithelial lining to cornified stratified squamous epithelium.

Etiology

- *Pseudomonas aeruginosa.*
- *Chlamydia psittasci.*
- *Mycoplasma bovigenitalium.*
- *Actinomyces pyogenes.*
- *Corynebacterium renale.*
- *Brucella abortus.*
- *E. coli.*

Macroscopic features

- Melanosis in bulbourethral glands.
- Enlargement/hardness of seminal vesicle.

Microscopic features

- Metaplasia of columnar epithelium into severely cornified stratified squamous epithelium.
- Proliferation of melanoblasts/melanocytes.

Prostatitis

Prostatitis is the inflammation of prostate gland by formation of painful abscess, atrophy, hyperplasia of epithelial cells, proliferation of fibroblasts and formation of cysts. It occurs in dogs.

Etiology

- Hormonal imbalance.
- Pyogenic staphylococci, streptococci.

Macroscopic features

- Presence of abscess encapsulated by fibrous tissue.
- Enlargement of prostate causing obstruction of urethra.
- Obstruction in rectal passage.
- Hematuria.

Microscopic features

- Infiltration of neutrophils and liquefied necrosis.
- Chronic inflammation is characterized by hyperplasia of glandular epithelium, fibroblasts and smooth muscle fibers.
- Cystic glandular hyperplasia.
- Infiltration of lymphocytes.

Balanoposthitis

Balanoposthitis is the inflammation of prepuce and glans penis characterized by phimosis or paraphimosis and pain during copulation. Balanitis is inflammation of glans penis and posthitis is inflammation of prepuce (Fig. 8.21).

A

B

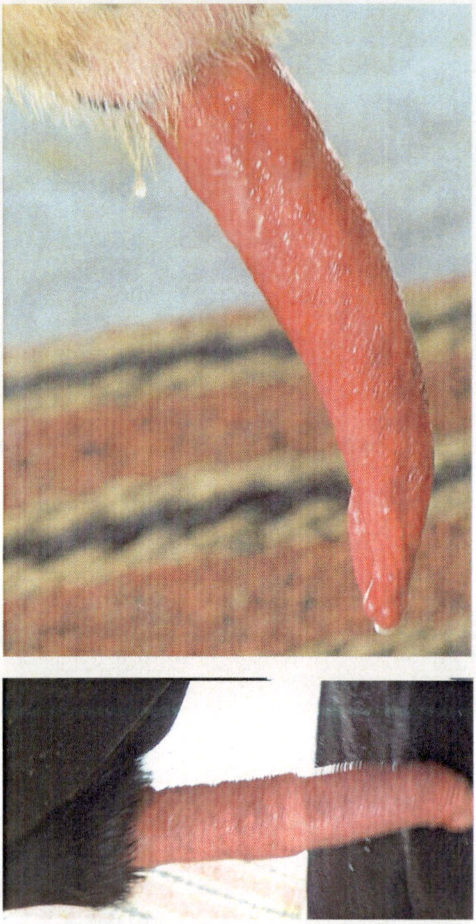

Fig. 8.21: Pustular balanoposthitis in a bull due to BHV-1 virus infection – pustules on penis (A and B)

Etiology

- *Trichomonas foetus*.
- BHV-1 virus.
- Vesicular exanthema virus.
- *Mycoplasma* spp.
- *Pseudomonas aeruginosa.*
- *Actinomyces pyogenes.*
- *Corynebacterium renale.*

Macroscopic features

- Phimosis and paraphimosis due to pain, adhesions.
- Congestion.

Microscopic features

- Fibrinopurulent exudate.
- Lymphocytic infiltration, congestion.

9

Pathology of Nervous System

Nervous system is composed of brain, spinal cord, and peripheral nerves. The neuron is a basic functional unit of nervous system. Necrosis of neurons in brain is known as encephalomalacia while necrosis of neurons in spinal cord is termed as myelomalacia. If the necrosis occurs in grey matter it is known as polioencephalomalacia while necrosis of neurons in white matter is called as leukoencephalomalacia. There are three types of scavenger cells in nervous system known as microglial, oligodendroglial and astrocytes. Microglial cells surround the necrotic neurons and are known as satellite cells and the process is called as satellitosis. As the neuron dies, it is engulfed by microglial cell and this process is termed as neuronophagia. The necrosis of nerve fibers starts from myelin sheath and this change is called demyelination or Wallerian degeneration.

The brain and spinal cord is covered by meninges. The inflammation of meninges is termed as meningitis. Meningoencephalitis is used for inflammation of both meninges and brain. Inflammation of duramater is known as pachymeningitis and of piamater is termed as leptomeningitis. Hydrocephalus means accumulation of clear fluid in ventricles and in sub arachnoid space due to obstruction in drainage. Hydrocephalus occurs in neonatal calves due to influenza and parainfluenza virus and is termed as congenital hydrocephalus.

Some nutritional deficiency like vitamin A, folic acid, vitamin B_{12}, niacin and zinc may also lead to hydrocephalus. Cerebeller hypoplasia has been observed due to bovine virus diarrhoea, hog cholera and feline panleukopenia virus. Some other congenital malformations are as under:

- Anencephaly means absence of brain.
- Microencephaly means small size of brain.
- Cranioschisis is failure of cranium to fuse which results in hernia of meninges known as meningocele.
- Hernia of meninges and brain is known as meningoencephalocele.

Encephalitis

Encephalitis is the inflammation of brain characterized by purulent/lymphocytic or proliferative changes. Encephalomyelitis is the inflammation of brain as well as spinal cord (Figs. 9.1 to 9.13).

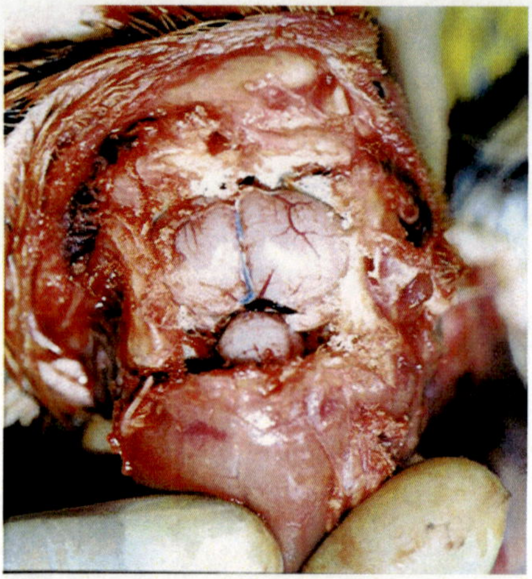

Fig. 9.1: Photograph of brain showing congestion in congestion in poultry

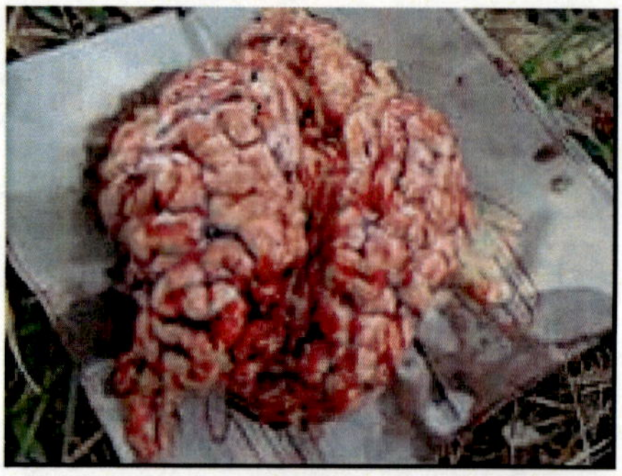

Fig. 9.2: Photograph in brain brain showing

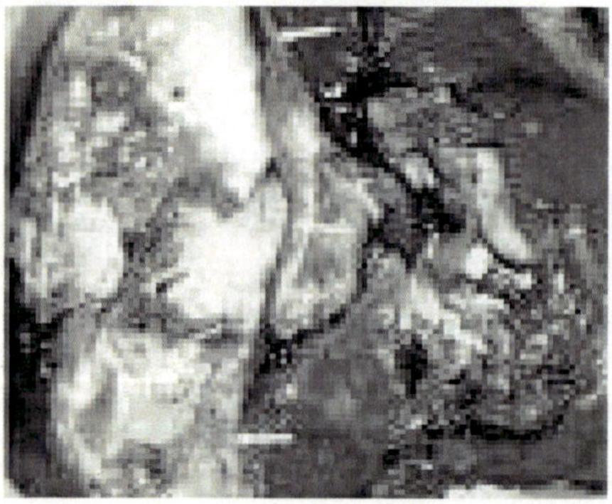

Fig. 9.3. Photograph showing abscess in brain BVD virus

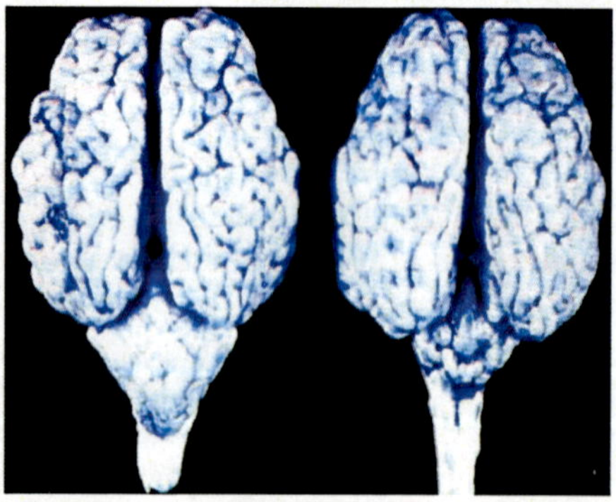

Fig. 9.4: Photograph of a calf showing cerebeller hypoplasia due to

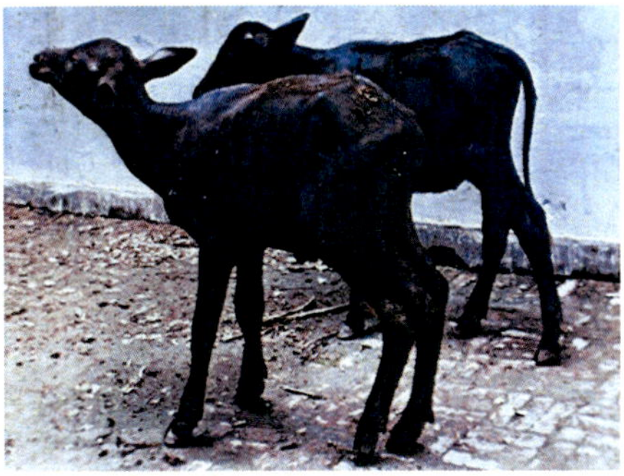

Fig. 9.5: Photograph showing staggering gait in buffalo calf due to strychnine poisoning

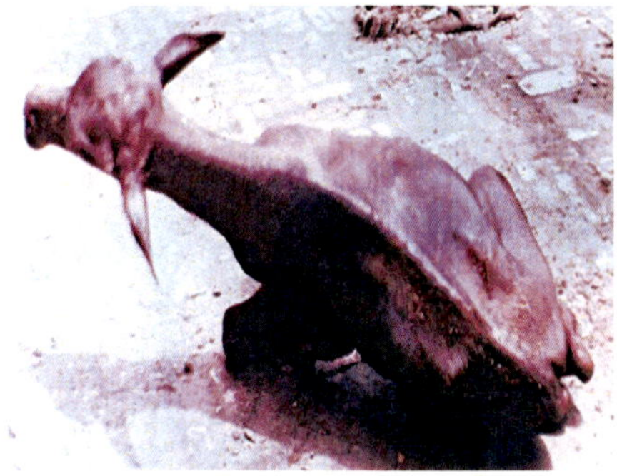

Fig. 9.6: Photograph showing spasms in neck due to strychnine poisoning

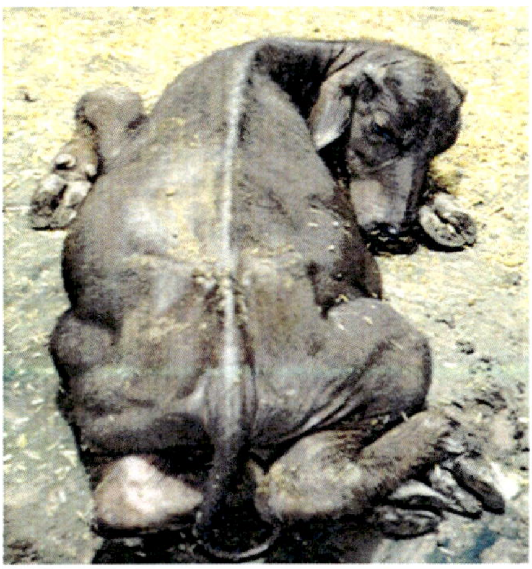

Fig. 9.7: Photograph showing torticollis in buffalo calf due to strychnine poisoning

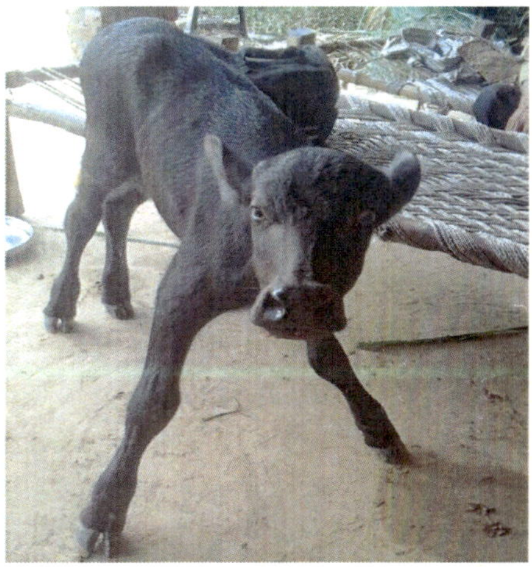

Fig. 9.8: Photograph showing nervous signs and stiffness of muscles.

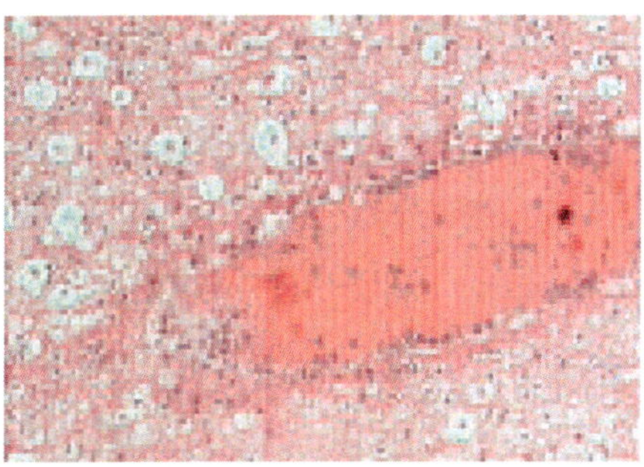

Fig. 9.9: Photomicrograph showing perivascular cuffing in brain.

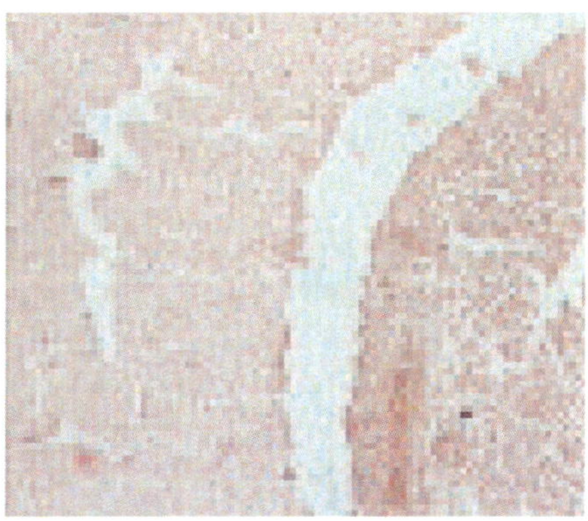

Fig. 9.10: Photomicrograph showing menigoencephalitis

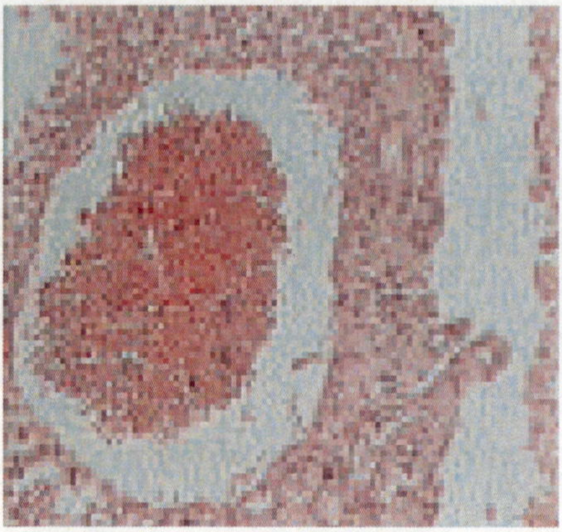

Fig. 9.11: Photomicrograph showing congestion and infiltration of inflammatory cells in brain

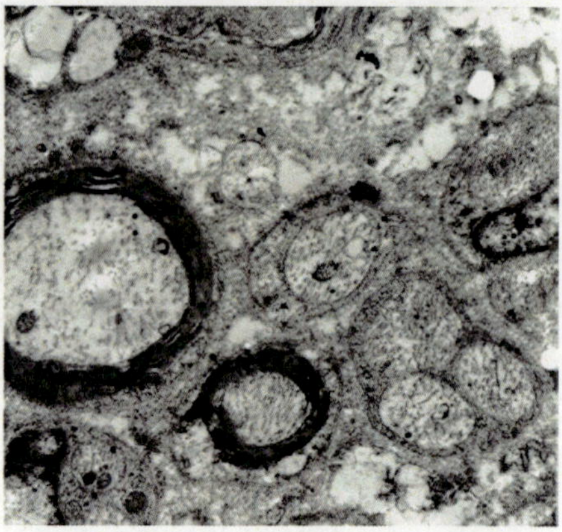

Fig. 9.12: Electron microphotograph of brain showing increase in endoneural space and Wallerian degeneration in nerve fiber.

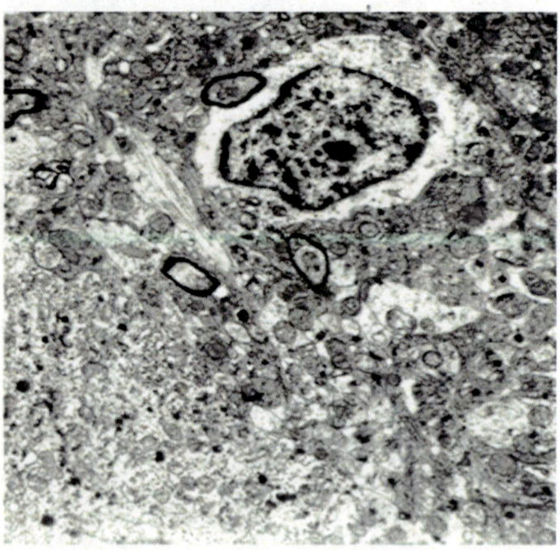

Fig. 9.13: Electron microphotograph of brain showing phagocytosis of degenerated nerve cell by phagocytic cell (Neuronophagia)

Etiology

- Bacteria
- *Listeria monocytogenes (L. ivanovii)* main cause
- *Haemophius* spp. *Pasturella* spp.
- Virus.
- Mycoplasma.
- Strychnine poisoning.

Macroscopic features

- Congestion.
- Hemorrhage.
- Small, tiny abscess.
- Necrosis also known as encephalomalacia.
- Involvement of spinal cord leads to encephalomyelitis and of meninges and is termed as meningoencephalitis.

Microscopic features

- Tiny or micro abscess in cerebrum.
- Infiltration by neutrophils and lymphocytes.
- Perivascular cuffing in Virchow Robin space by lymphocytes.
- Necrosis of neurons.
- Satellitosis, neuronophagia.
- Pleocytosis- Increase in number of white blood cells in cerebrospinal fluid.

Encephalomalacia

Encephalomalacia is the necrosis of nervous tissue in brain characterized by loss of normal architecture and soft friable liquefied mass (Figs. 9.14 & 9.15).

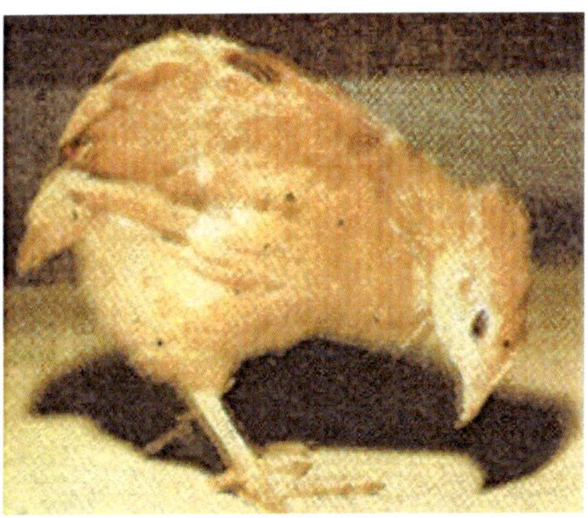

Fig. 9.14: Photograph showing encephalomalacia in a chick

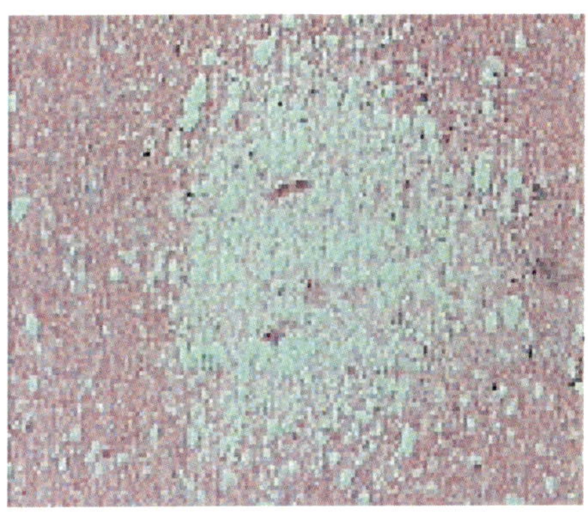

Fig. 9.15: Photomicrograph showing encephalomalacia

Etiology

- Deficiency of copper, thiamine, vitamin E.
- Poisons: Bracken fern, lead, mercury, salt poisoning, enterotoxaemia, mycotoxins.

Macroscopic features

- Encephalomalacia - necrosis in brain.
- Myelomalacia - necrosis in spinal cord.
- Poliomalacia - necrosis in brain gray matter.
- Leukomalacia - necrosis in brain white matter.
- Soft, friable liquefied mass in brain.
- Congestion.

Microscopic features

- Liquefactive necrosis.
- Surrounded by neurological cells/scavenger cells.
- Proliferation of small new capillaries

Spongiform Encephalopathy

Spongiform encephalopathy is characterized by the presence of vacuoles in grey and/or white matter.

Etiology

- Prion proteins.
- Scrapie in sheep.
- BSE in cattle.

Macroscopic features

- No characteristic gross lesion.
- Oedema of brain or hydrocephalus.
- Congestion.

Microscopic features

- Vacuolation in white and grey matter.
- Vacuoles are usually in neurons, glial cells and in myelin.
- Vacuoles are more extensive in medulla, pons and mid brain and give brain "spongy form".

Meningitis

Meningitis is the inflammation of meninges, usually occurs along with encephalitis or encephalomyelitis and is characterized by congestion and infiltration of neutrophils and mononuclear cells. Pachymeningitis is inflammation of dura mater while leptomenigitis involves the pia mater.

Etiology

- Virus e.g. swine fever.
- Trauma.
- Bacteria e.g. Pasturella, Listeria.
- Toxoplasma.
- Leptospira.

Macroscopic features

- Congestion.
- Thickening of meninges.
- Petechial hemorrhage.

Microscopic features

- Congestion.
- Infiltration of neutrophils and lymphocytes.
- Fibrosis.

Neuritis

Neuritis is the inflammation of nerves along with degenerative changes characterized by oedema, infiltration of inflammatory cells (Fig. 9.16 to 9.18).

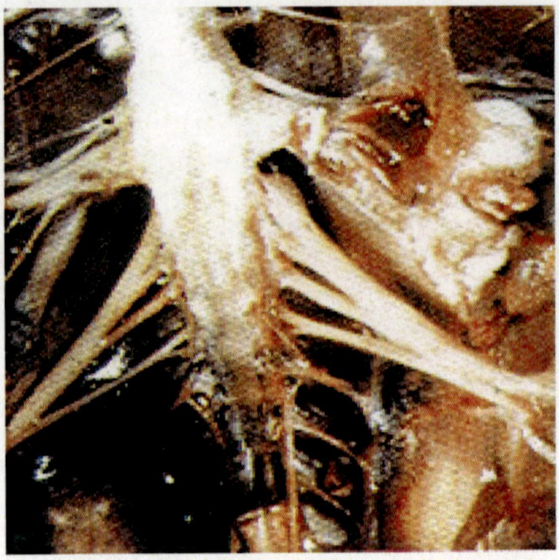

Fig. 9.16: Photograph showing neuritis due to Marek's disease

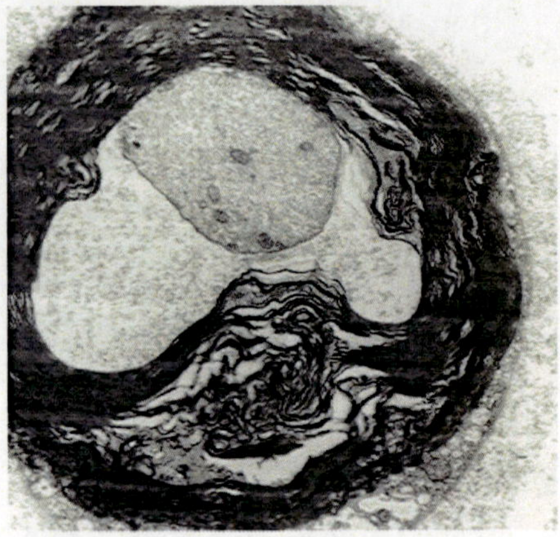

Fig. 9.17: Fig. 9.17: Electron microphotograph of sciatic nerve showing degeneration of myelinated fibres with swelling and fragmentation

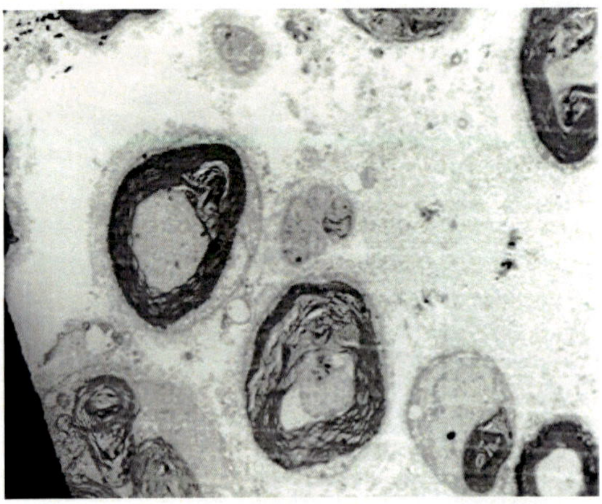

Fig. 9.18: Electron microphotograph of sciatic nerve showing advanced Wallerian degeneration and increased endoneural space.

Etiology

- Toxins.
- Trauma.
- Virus e.g. Marek's disease MD.
- Lead and Mercury.

- Bacteria e.g. Strangles.
- Deficiency of vitamin E.

Macroscopic features

- No characteristic gross lesion.
- Oedema of nerve.

Microscopic features

- Wallerian degeneration.
- Infiltration of neutrophils and lymphocytes.
- More destruction at distal end of the neuron.

10

Pathology of Endocrine System, Eyes and Ear

Pathology of Endocrine System

Pathology of Hypothalamus

The lesions in hypothalamus may cause diabetes insipidus characterized by polydipsia and polyuria with low specific gravity of urine. It occurs due to deficiency of antidiuretic hormone vasopressin.

Etiology/ Occurrence

- Lesions in hypothalamus and/or pituitary.
- Adenoma and adenocarcinoma of pituitary.
- Necrosis of hypothalamic nuclei due to larval migration.

Pathology of Pituitary Gland

Hyperpituitarism

Hyperpituitarism is increased secretion of hormone(s) from pituitary gland such as excessive secretion of somatotropic hormone which may cause gigantism characterized by increased length of long bones, heavy and thick bones leading to large hands, feet, skull bones (acromegaly). Hyperpituitarism also increases adrenal cortical stimulating hormone leading to hyperplasia of adrenal cortex. Pituitary adenoma or adeno-carcinoma is responsible for hyperpituitarism.

Hypopituitarism

Hypopituitarism is decrease in pituitary hormone secretions due to atrophy, aplasia or hypoplasia of pituitary. Systemic diseases such as meningitis of bacterial or viral origin may also cause lesions in pituitary e.g. infectious canine hepatitis, hog cholera. It is characterized by dwarfism, genital hypoplasia and prolonged gestation period.

Pathology of Thyroid

Hyperthyroidism

Hyperthyroidism is increased activity of thyroid gland leading to increased production of thyroxin characterized by tachycardia, increased basal metabolic rate, bulging of eyeballs and early maturity. It occurs due to presence of tumor in thyroid. Other signs include polydipsia, polyuria, and loss of weight, weakness, fatigue and hyperthermia.

Hypothyroidism

Hypothyroidism is reduced activity of thyroid gland characterized by decreased basal metabolic rate, obesity, retardation of growth and sexual development leading to cretinism. In adult, it is characterized by myxomatous mucoid degeneration in subcutaneous region giving floppy and oedematous appearance. Hypothyroidism is caused by aplasia or hypoplasia of thyroid gland.

Goiter

Goiter is enlargement of thyroid gland, which may be accompanied by hypo- or hyperthyroidism. The enlargement of thyroid is due to hyperplasia, inflammation, or proliferation of connective tissue. The hyperplasia of gland is characterized by increased height and number to epithelial cells in acini of gland. It may be caused by deficiency of iodine, thiouracil toxicity and by use of goiterogenic substances such as soybean and cabbage. The goiter has been classified into 6 forms described as under:

Hyperplastic goiter

Due to iodine deficiency, there is hyperplasia of thyroid gland with reduction in thyroxin production. It occurs due to increased level of thyrotropic hormone from pituitary gland.

Familial goiter

There is hyperplasia of thyroid gland with reduced thyroxin secretion caused by defective or absence of enzymes responsible for thyroxin synthesis. It is not related with iodine deficiency but has congenital basis of occurrence

Colloid goiter

Colloid goiter is enlargement and distention of acini filled with colloid and flat epithelium caused by deficiency of iodine.

Adenomatous goiter

This is characterized by nodular enlargement of thyroid gland, with one or many hard nodules of variable size and characteristic adenoma of gland.

Toxic goiter

Toxic goiter is characterized by exophthalmus due to hyperthyroidism, enlargement of thyroid due to hyperplasia, and occurs as a hypersecretion of thyrotropic hormone from pituitary.

Equine goiter

Equine goiter is caused by excessive iodine levels in feed and occurs in new born foals with weakness from a goiterous mare. These foals have enlarged thyroid gland.

Lymphocytic Thyroditis

Lymphocytic thyroditis is characterized by infiltration of lymphocytes in gland causing destruction and is caused by autoimmune mechanism. The infiltration of lymphocytes is so severe that it gives lymphofollicular appearance.

Pathology of Parathyroid Gland

Hypoparathyroidism

Hypoparathyroidism is decreased activity of parathyroid gland characterized by decreased concentration of blood calcium and tonic spasms of muscles. It occurs due to infection, neoplasms, low calcium diets and hypersecretion of thyrocalcitonin.

Hyperparathyroidism

Hyperparathyroidism is the increased activity of parathyroid gland characterized by weakness, polydipsia, polyuria, hypercalcemia nephrocalcinosis, demineralization of bones, metastatic calcification in soft tissues and fibrous osteodystrophy. It may occur in adenoma or adenocarcinoma of parathyroid and hyperplasia of gland. Hyperparathyroidism is also associated with renal disease and chronic hypocalcemia and produces more parathormone hormone.

Pathology of Adenal Glands

Hypoadrenocorticism

Hypoadrenocorticism is decreased activity of adrenal cortex characterized by atrophy, necrosis and decreased hormones leading to low blood pressure, decreased blood volume, hypoglycemia, gastrointestinal malfunction and hyperpigmentation in skin. It may occur in tuberculosis, histoplasmosis, amyloidosis, neoplasms and drug toxicity.

Hyperadrenocorticism

Hyperadrenocorticism is increased activity of adrenal cortex characterized by hyperplasia and neoplasia of the gland leading to alopecia, muscle weakness, pendulous abdomen, obesity, polyuria, polydipsia, lymphopenia, eosinophilia, neutrophilia and excessive secretion of 17- ketogenic steroids.

Pathology of Pancreas

Pancreatic islets or islets of Langerhans' are responsible for production of insulin, deficiency of which may cause hyperglycemia or diabetes mellitus. It is characterized by polyuria, glycosuria, hyperglycemia, polydipsia, loss of secretory granules in β-cells of pancreatic islets. It is caused by inflammation of pancreas causing exocrine pancreatitis. This condition may lead to arteriosclerosis in blood vessels of animals.

Pathology of Pineal Gland

The pineal gland is responsible for secretion of melatonin hormone which inhibits gonadotropic hormone synthesis and release by pituitary and thus plays an important role in seasonal estrus/reproductive capacity of animals. Degeneration and necrosis of gland may cause its decreased function but it is not well reported. Adenoma of gland may be associated with increased sexual libido and activity.

Pathology of Eye

Blepheritis is the inflammation of eyelids while the term conjunctivitis is used to describe the inflammatory condition of conjunctiva and keratitis for cornea. In ward turning of eyelid is known as entropion which may result in keratitis or conjunctivitis. Conjunctivitis is also caused by double row of eye lashes (disctichiasis).

Developmental Anomalies

- Aphakia is the absence of lens.
- Microphakia is the small size of lens.
- Hypoplasia of optic nerve is underdeveloped optic nerve with absence of optic nerve layer and ganglion cell layer of retina.

- Agenesis of optic nerve is absence of optic nerve.
- Coloboma is the congenital defect in the continuity of one of the tunics of the eye i.e. iris.
- Congenital anophthalmos is the absence of the eye which may occur due to vitamin A deficiency in dam.
- Congenital microphathalmos is the decreased size of eyes and may occur due to maternal vitamin A deficiency
- Congenital opacity of cornea occurs in cattle and dogs due to effect of inherited recessive gene trait.
- Hemeralopia is day blindness which may occur in dogs due to single autosomal recessive gene.

Keratoconjunctivitis

Keratoconjunctivitis is the inflammation of cornea and conjunctiva characterized by congestion of eyes, blindness, opacity and corneal oedema (Figs 10.1 to 10.9).

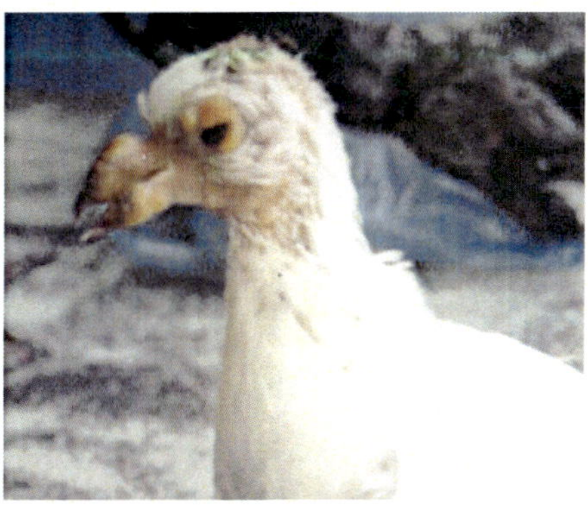

Fig. 10.1: Photograph showing conjunctivitis in pigeon due to poxvirus infection

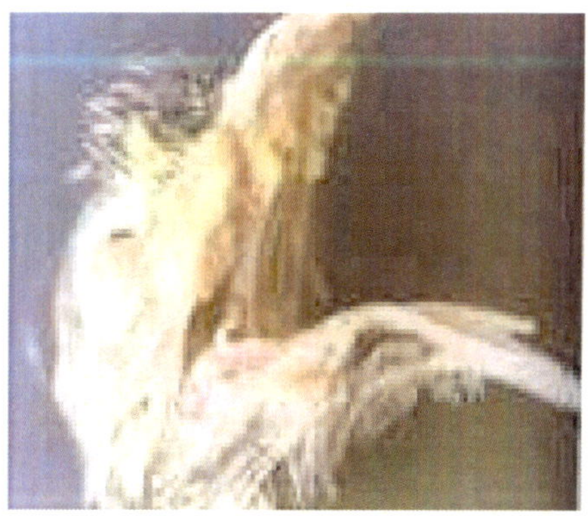

Fig. 10.2: Photograph showing conjunctivitis in pigeon due to poxvirus infection

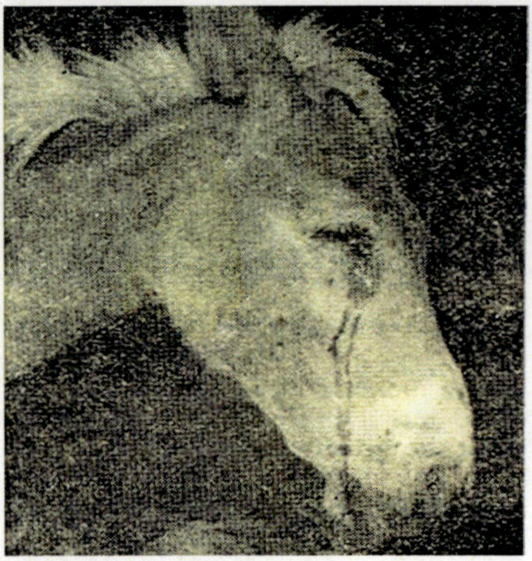

Fig. 10.3: Photograph showing mucopurulant discharge from eyes due to mallein test in horse

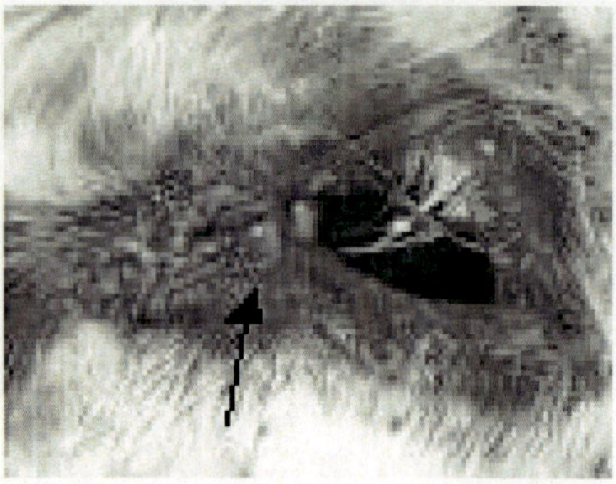

Fig.10.4: Photograph showing mucopurulant exudate in eye

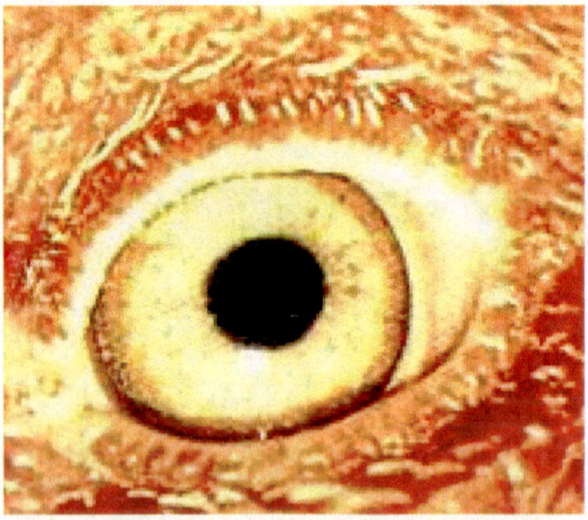

Fig. 10.5: Photograph showing iridocyclitis

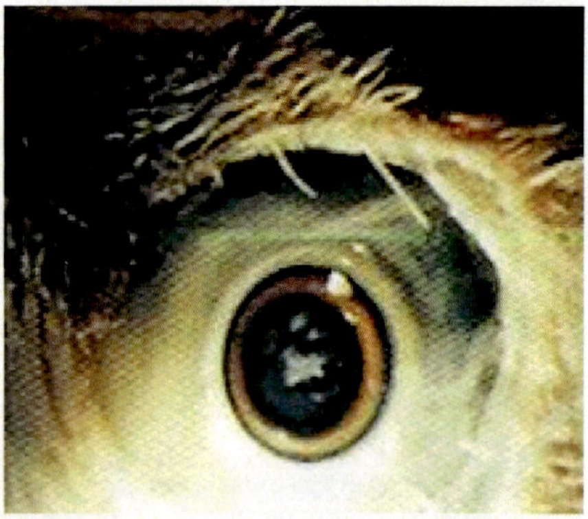

Fig. 10.6: Photograph showing cataract

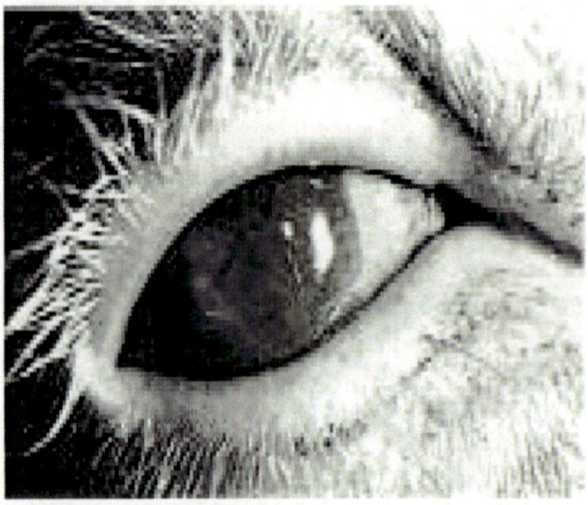

Fig. 10.7: Photograph showing corneal opacity

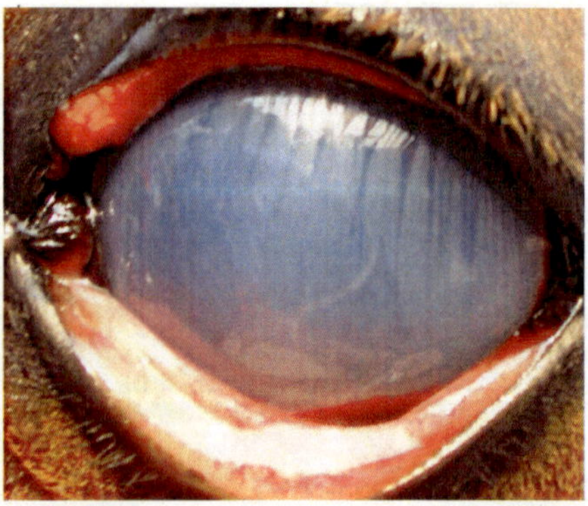

Fig. 10.8: Photograph showing presence of parasite in eye.

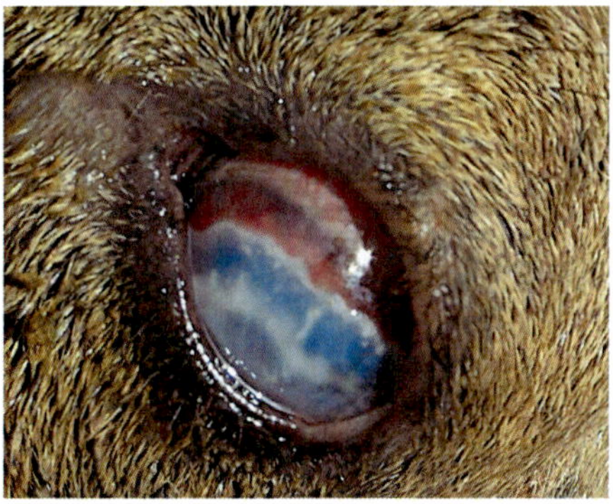

Fig. 10.9: Photograph of eye showing corneal opacity.

Etiology

- Penetrating foreign objects e.g. Awns of wheat.
- *Moraxella bovis.*
- *Mycoplasma* spp.
- BHV-1, poxvirus.
- *Rickettsia conjunctivae.*
- *Chlamydia* spp.
- spp.
- Allergy.

Macroscopic features

- Congestion of conjunctiva leading to redness "pink eye".
- Oedema, pain
- Increased lacrimation (decreased lacrimation also causes conjunctivitis).
- Corneal opacity.

Cataract

Cataract is opacity of lens and is classified as under:

- Subcapsular cataract is the opacity of lens due to abnormal proliferation of lens epithelium in anterior end as a result of injury.
- Posterior polar cataract is opacity of lens due to abnormal growth of lens epithelium at posterior face of lens

- Cortical cataract is opacity of lens due to disorganization of the lens fibres.
- Nuclear cataract is the increased density of fibres of lens at the centre and occurs in old animals.
- Morgagnian cataract is the liquefaction of cortical substance and has not been observed in animals.
- Congenital cataract is seen in neonatal animals and occurs due to failure of closure of primary lens vesicle at the periphery of lens vesicle and is associated with chediak - Higashi Syndrome.

Retinitis

Retinitis is the inflammation of retina caused by trauma, iritis, iridocyclitis and choroiditis. When it is associated with inflammation of choroids, it is known as chorioretinitis. It may lead to detachment of retina. Iritis is inflammation of iris. Iridocyclitis is the inflammation of iris and uvea. Choroiditis is inflammation of choroid plexus.

The chorioretinitis is characterized by glaucoma occurs in canine distemper, feline panleukopenia, toxoplasmosis, tuberculosis, coccidioidomycosis, deficiency of vitamin A and bracken fern poisoning.

Glaucoma

Glaucoma is the intraoccular hypertension due to occlusion of the filtration angle and is caused by trauma, iridocyclitis, intraoccular hemorrhage and neoplasm. It may be unilateral or bilateral. It is characterized by enlargement of eye ball, opaque cornea and increase aqueous humor.

Pathology of Ear

Otitis Externa

Otitis externa is inflammation of external ear caused by *Actinomyces bovis*, parasites and fungus and characterized by granulomatous inflammation (Fig. 10.10).

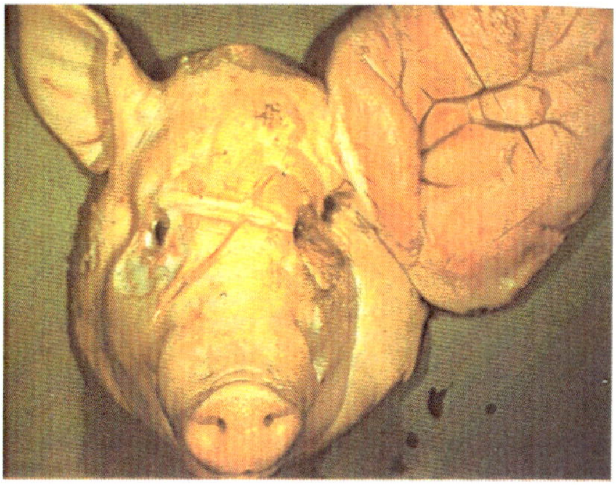

Fig. 10.10: Photograph showing otitis externa in pig.

Etiology

- *Actinomyces bovis.*
- *Psoroptes communis* – mite.
- *Otobius megnini* – tick.
- Fungi – (otomycosis).
- Grass of wheat awns.

Macroscopic features

- Swelling and congestion leading to obstruction of ear canal.
- Excessive production of thick, tenacious and brownish wax.
- Granulomatous lesions filling the external auditory meatus

Microscopic features

- Granulomatous lesions of actinomycosis in subcutaneous region around the cartilage.

Otitis Media

Otitis media is inflammation of middle ear including tympanic cavity and eustachian tube.

Etiology

- Infections from otitis externa or nasopharynx.
- Mites.

- Awns of wheat.
- *Pasteurella* spp.

Macroscopic features

- Occlusion of eustachian tube.
- Purulent inflammation.

Microscopic features

- Suppurative inflammation.

Otitis Interna

Otitis interna is the inflammation of inner ear including membranous and osseous labyrinth. This is also known as labyrinthitis.

Etiology

- Infection from otitis media.
- *Mycoplasma* spp.
- Mumps.
- Measles.

Macroscopic features

- Disturbance in equilibrium.
- Deafness.

Microscopic features

- Suppurative inflammation.

Index

H

I

K

L

R

S

T